THE
weed gummies
COOKBOOK

**RECIPES FOR CANNABIS CANDIES,
THC & CBD EDIBLES, AND MORE**

AUTHOR & PHOTOGRAPHER

monica lo

"Lo covers it all without wasting any kief: all the ways and whys of infusion; the options for tools and techniques at every level of cooking experience; the cultural and personal context behind these sweets. The recipes span nostalgic flavors and textures, offering satisfying takes on classics and inventive delicacies influenced by her explorations of Asian culinary heritage. *The Weed Gummies Cookbook* is an essential guide to infused sweets at home, as well as a testament to the way this plant creates space for people to more creatively explore their culture and passions."

—Lauren Yoshiko

Cannabis journalist and contributor at *Broccoli Mag* and *Thrillist*

"Demystifying the process of creating cannabis confections, *The Weed Gummies Cookbook* will empower you to make your own gummies, caramels, and hard candies. Learn how to estimate THC dosages, infuse sugars and fats, and experiment with unique recipes featuring sophisticated flavors and techniques. Follow Lo's expert advice and you'll never need to visit a dispensary again!"

—Elise McDonough

Author of *The Official High Times Cannabis Cookbook*

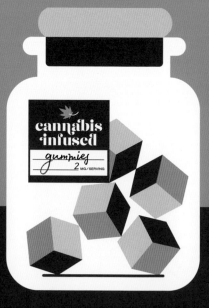

Published by:
ULYSSES PRESS
PO Box 3440
Berkeley, CA 94703
www.ulyssespress.com

ISBN: 978-1-64604-366-8
Library of Congress Control Number: 2022932304

Printed in China
10 9 8 7 6 5 4 3

Acquisitions editor: Casie Vogel
Managing editor: Claire Chun
Project editor: Renee Rutledge
Editor: Anne Healey
Proofreader: Michele Anderson
Design and layout: Monica Lo
Photograph page 126: Heather Tafolla
Production: Winnie Liu

NOTE TO READERS:
This book has been written and published strictly for informational and educational purposes
only. It is not intended to serve as medical advice or to be any form of medical treatment.
You should always consult your physician before altering or changing any aspect of your
medical treatment and/or undertaking a diet regimen, including the guidelines described
in this book. Do not stop or change any prescription medications without the guidance or
advice of your physician. Any use of the information in this book is made on the reader's good
judgment after consulting with his or her physician and is the reader's sole responsibility. This
book is not intended to diagnose or treat any medical condition and is not a substitute for
a physician. The author and publisher disclaim liability for any medical outcomes that may
occur as a result of applying the methods suggested in this book. This book is independently
authored and published, and no sponsorship or endorsement of this book by and no
affiliation with, any trademarked brands or other products mentioned within is claimed. All
trademarked brands that appear in ingredient lists and elsewhere in this book belong to
their respective owners and are used here for informational purposes only. The author and
publisher encourage readers to patronize the quality brands mentioned in this book.

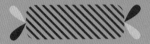

FOR MY SWEETIES

david & milo

contents

2 soft caramels & nougats

3 hard & brittle

4 sugar alternatives

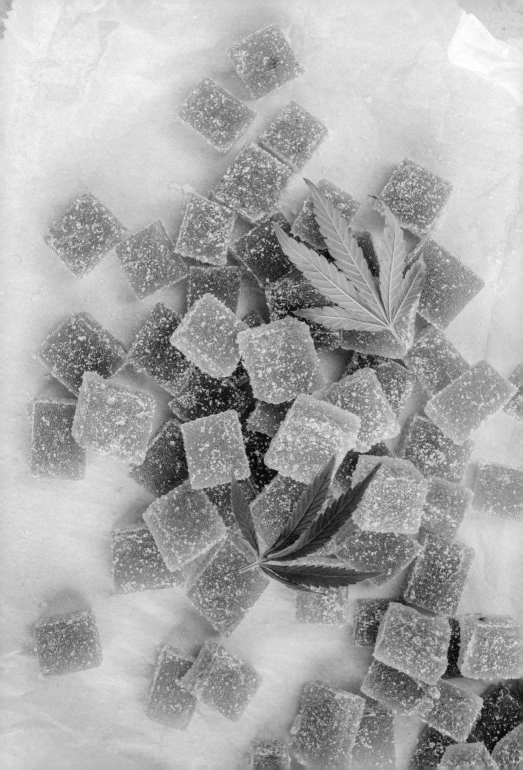

preface

I often think about how I ended up where I am today, and I'm amazed at how much it's been shaped by cannabis. My journey pivoted in 2015 when I naïvely joined a high-intensity bootcamp workout with my then boyfriend (who is now my husband.) I herniated a spinal disk within the first week of class.

My doctor prescribed a mixture of opioids and acetaminophen, but my adverse reactions to these, on top of the chronic back pain, were too much to handle. In desperate need of relief, I tried the cannabis-infused treats my roommate offered to me. And for the first time in a long time, I slept like a baby. The next day, I found myself spending hours upon hours researching this plant and how to make my own infusions.

Since we lived in a strict no-smoking building, I needed to be very discreet with the wafting scent of cannabis; this meant that using a Crock-Pot or cooking on the stovetop was not in the cards. At the time I was a creative director of a sous vide start-up and thought I'd put our machines to the test; thus, *Sous Weed®* was born.

Sous vide *(pronounced sue-veed)* refers to the process of placing your food in a sealed bag or airtight jar and cooking it in a pot of water at a very precise temperature. Since the cannabis and oil are sealed up and placed underwater to infuse—there's no smell! With a sous vide machine, there's no need to babysit an open flame. You can walk away and go about your day without worrying about overcooking your cannabis.

Feeding people has always been my love language. I was excited to test my creations on friends and share my recipes online. Documenting my sous vide cannabis experiments not only helped me manage my back pain in a less invasive manner but also kept me in a positive and creative headspace.

Deep-diving into history, I was shocked to discover that the medicinal properties of cannabis were first recorded in *Pen Ts'ao*, a Chinese pharmacological book written in the second century. Shen Nong, the father of Chinese herbal medicine, had documented various classifications of cannabis, which suggests that the Chinese had a special relationship with the plant. Hemp seeds were used in breakfast porridges because they're a powerhouse of energy and fiber; cannabis flower was used to help with seizures and insomnia as well as to promote female wellness. Not only was cannabis regarded as a foundational herb in ancient Chinese medicine, but it was also widely used in Hong Kong, Taiwan, Japan, South Korea, and India. This is just a really long way to say that cannabis use can be traced back to the beginning of documented history.

With immense love for this plant and an urge to reconnect with my roots, I cofounded Asian Americans for Cannabis Education with my two partners in 2015 to start a dialogue about the stigmatization of cannabis and legalization among Asian American communities. In 2019 I had the honor of presenting my studies on cannabis in ancient Asia at the Asian Art Museum in San Francisco.

Cannabis has since become the intersection of my passions and skills. It has opened doors for me to collaborate with farmers, cannabis entrepreneurs, chefs, and edibles makers to build brands, develop recipes, and create art.

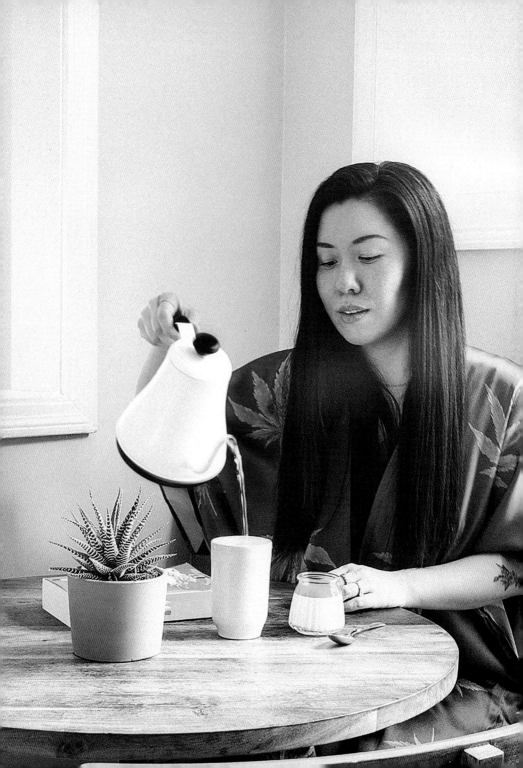

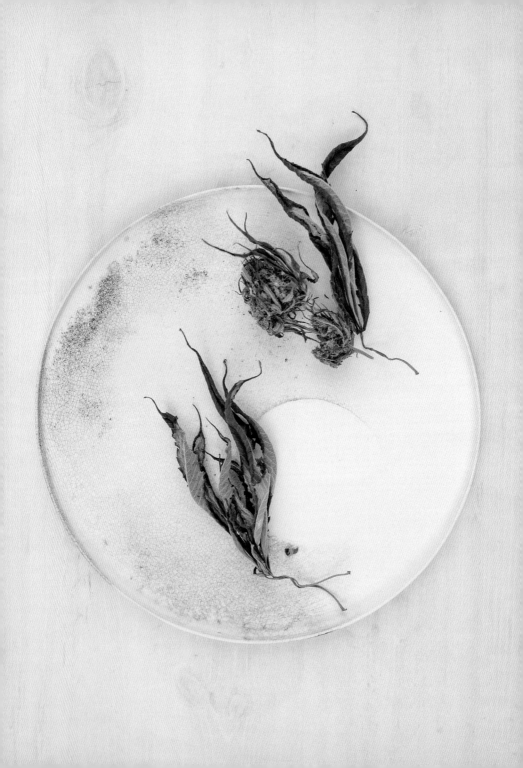

ethos

Sous Weed, my educational blog, is proudly Asian American owned and female led. While the platform is driven by food content, the soul of the work is committed to advocating for the legalization and decriminalization of cannabis as well as promoting equity in our industry.

It's important for us all to be thoughtful cannabis consumers and to understand where the products we consume come from. Supporting drug policy reform and cannabis criminal justice reform work is also crucial. There are far too many people still incarcerated for nonviolent cannabis offenses while others are building immense wealth off this plant. The "Educational Resources" section of this book (page 116) will give you access to cannabis educators, a database of BIPOC-owned businesses to shop at, and nonprofit organizations to support.

A portion of the profits from *The Weed Gummies Cookbook* will be donated semiannually to the Last Prisoner Project.

introduction

Cannabis edibles, specifically gummies and sweet confections, have seen increasing popularity over the past few years. One impact of the COVID-19 pandemic was that many consumers made the switch to edibles, opting to refrain from inhalable forms of consumption. Edibles sales in medical and recreational state markets saw immense growth in 2020 and 2021, spurring on a new age of innovative cannabis treats and beverages.

With more medical patients, the canna-curious, and mature consumers now gaining legal access to cannabis, there is higher demand for delicious infused goods. Cannabis edibles have a low barrier to entry (everyone eats!) and are easy to introduce into your everyday lifestyle.

But let's be frank. If you live in a state with legal cannabis access, you are probably experiencing higher prices due to licensing costs, operating expenses, and taxes. Edibles, oils, flower, and tinctures are becoming increasingly expensive, which means consumers are finding it difficult to get cannabis products at affordable prices and in the dosages they need.

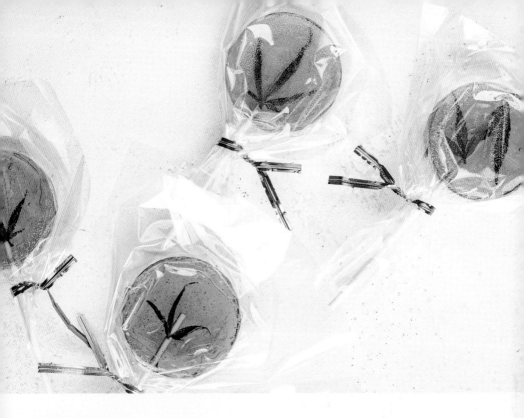

why diy?

The main reason for DIY is that it's far more cost-effective to make your infusions and treats at home, especially as dispensary prices skyrocket. You are also not limited to what the shop has in stock.

- You can get strain-specific or phytocannabinoid-specific cannabis and use your favorite flower.

- It allows you to customize your dose to your body's needs.

- Treats can be made healthier without preservatives.

- You can create extra-special gifts for family and friends during the holidays.

This user-friendly cookbook is designed to build your culinary cannabis repertoire and help you feel empowered to make your edibles at home.

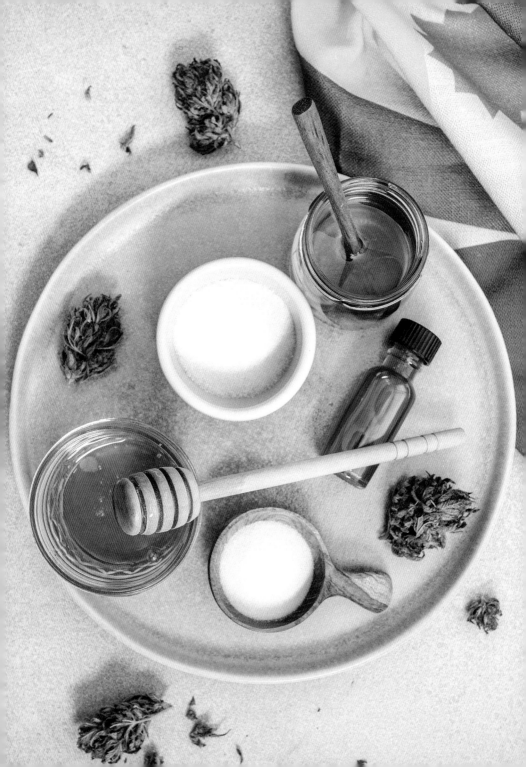

THE
cannabis confections pantry

Most of the ingredients for the recipes in this cookbook can be found in your local grocery store, an Asian supermarket, or even online. When you can, grab your fresh produce from a farmers' market because it will always taste better than store-bought.

cannabis & hemp

Hemp and cannabis are the same plant! So what's the difference? Hemp contains 0.3 percent or less tetrahydrocannabinol (THC), while cannabis contains more than 0.3 percent THC. Cannabidiol (CBD) can be derived from both these plants. There are over 100 phytocannabinoids (plant-derived cannabinoids that act on receptors in the endocannabinoid system), identified so far in the cannabis plant—THC and CBD being the two most notable. Hemp is federally legal under the 2018 Farm Bill. And as of 2021, the legality of cannabis varies state by state.

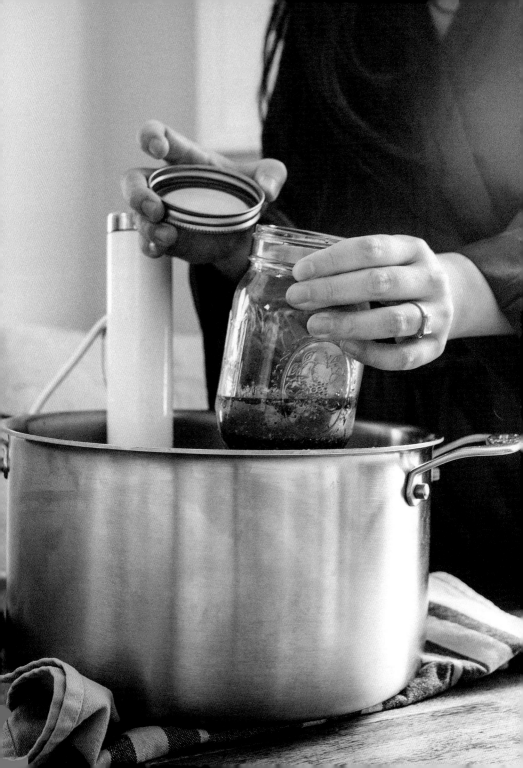

fats

Cannabis is fat and alcohol soluble. There are so many unique infusions you can make, but in this book we will focus on butter, medium-chain triglycerides (MCT) oil, and coconut oil.

tinctures

Cannabis tinctures can be made using high-proof alcohol, such as Everclear or another strong grain alcohol.

emulsifiers

Lecithin, a phosopholipid found in food, is used in certain recipes to help emulsify cannabis-infused fats with a water-based mixture. Sunflower lecithin is my preference because of its additional health benefits. It's also used as a supplement to prevent plugged milk ducts while breastfeeding!

sweeteners

Various sweeteners are used throughout this book. Some are used for color or textural purposes. Others, such as corn syrup, are used as an interferent, which helps prevent sugars from crystallizing and getting crusty on the surface of your gummies. Corn syrup is also used to create a more authentic commercial gummy texture. The "Sugar Alternatives" chapter contains recipes using unrefined sugar and natural sugar replacements.

gelatins & starches

Grass-fed gelatin is a natural protein made from the collagen in animal parts. It can be purchased in sheets or as a powder. All recipes tested in this cookbook use Vital Proteins Beef Gelatin in powdered form. Gelatin must first bloom in cold liquid for a few minutes before being added to a warm liquid to dissolve. Bloomed powdered gelatin will hydrate and swell into a clump. Keep in mind that high boiling temperatures will denature the gelatin.

Agar-agar is a strong gelling agent derived from red algae, making it a great vegan gelatin substitute. Texturally, it sets more firmly and has a crisper bite compared to grass-fed gelatin. It also comes in various forms, but for ease and accessibility, all agar-agar recipes in this cookbook use the Telephone brand powdered version, which can be found in most Asian supermarkets or online. Unlike gelatin, agar-agar needs to be brought to a boil for a few minutes to activate.

Pectin is a natural thickener extracted from fruits like apples or citrus and is primarily used in jams and jellies. In this cookbook, a rapid-set high-methoxyl (HM) pectin in powdered form is used in recipes with a higher acidity content.

Tapioca flour is a gluten-free starch derived from the cassava root. It's used in various Asian cakes and confections. It's also the main ingredient of the beloved bubble tea!

Cornstarch is a staple in my pantry. It's often used as a thickener in sauces, soups, and extra-crispy deep-fry batter. In candy making, it's an invaluable ingredient that will help dry and cure your gummies to create a firmer texture. A light dusting will also keep your candies from sticking to each other in humid weather.

food coloring

A small handful of recipes call for the optional food coloring. You can also get creative and swap the food coloring with a dash of fresh, colorful juice from fruit or greens like spinach or raw cannabis leaves.

cannabis infusion & candy equipment

- Silicone candy molds
- Silicone spatula
- Candy or instant-read thermometer
- Liquid measuring cup with spout
- Digital scale
- Heavy-bottomed saucepan in small, medium, and large sizes
- Double boiler
- 8-inch square baking pan
- Decarboxylator (such as the Ardent FX)
- Sous vide machine
- Heat-resistant kitchen gloves
- Fine-mesh strainer
- Candy funnel or candy dropper
- Silicone mat and/or parchment paper
- Baking sheet
- Candy-wrapping materials and stickers
- Silica gel desiccant packs to keep candies dry

safety & dosages

candy-making tips and safety notes

Before you dive right into the recipes, here are a few safety tips for using this book.

1. Read the recipe all the way through before you begin to cook. Some processes will require quick action so reviewing ahead will better prepare you for what's to come.

2. Controlling sugar temperature is a science! A candy thermometer is going to be your best friend for many of the recipes, especially in the "Hard & Brittle" chapter, which I've dubbed "The Danger Zone." Caramel burns are savage and heat-resistant kitchen gloves will come in handy as you transfer molten sugar into candy molds.

3. Special equipment will be listed with each recipe. Sugar work is finicky so a heavy-bottom stainless-steel or copper saucepan is crucial in the "Soft Caramels & Nougats" and "Hard & Brittle" chapters. Small-, medium-, and large-size saucepans will be noted in the recipes. When shopping for saucepans, opt for narrow and tall; it's also nice to find one with a pouring lip.

4. If humidity is an issue where you live, toss a small silica gel desiccant packet into the airtight container when you store your treats. This will help absorb moisture and keep your candies dry.

5. Practice makes perfect! If a recipe sounds challenging, try a test round first without your cannabis infusion to see how you fare. I have burnt many batches of caramel during my testing due to different variables and situations in the kitchen. It always pains me to toss out a batch that's been infused with the green goodness.

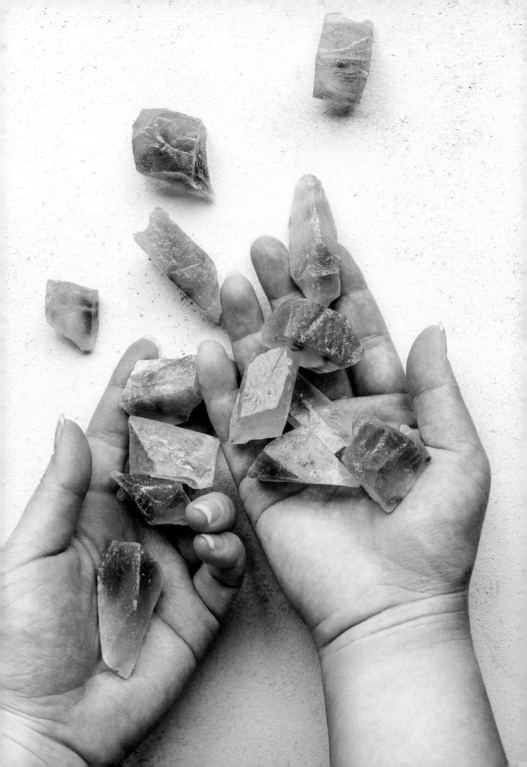

childproofing & labeling

Cannabis-infused treats need to be kept out of the reach of children. These candies may look tempting, so my advice is to purchase childproof jars and store homemade goods in a locked location or high on a shelf.

Be bold, bright, and direct with a cannabis warning label on all your packaging, especially when gifting infused confections to family and friends.

To prevent overconsumption of your delicious treats, please refer to the dosage estimation chart on page 27 to help you calculate the dosage.

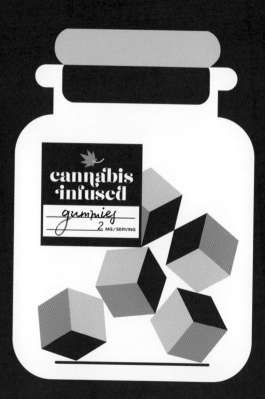

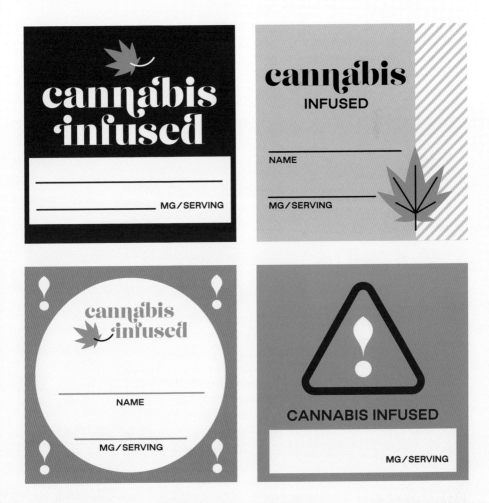

cannabis infused

_____

_____ MG/SERVING

cannabis
INFUSED

_____
NAME

_____
MG/SERVING

cannabis infused

_____
NAME

_____
MG/SERVING

CANNABIS INFUSED

MG/SERVING

Download and print these free customizable warning labels at SousWeed.com/Safety

cannabis edibles safety

"Start low and go slow" is a saying we often hear in our industry. These are wise words for the cannabis curious. Most state policies have legally set dispensary-bought edibles at 10 mg of THC for a single serving. For some individuals, that's far too much; for others, not nearly enough. Our bodies are unique, and we all metabolize cannabinoids differently, which is why I like to recommend trying a 2 mg to 5 mg dose to get a sense of how your own body reacts to a particular infusion or edible and then waiting up to two hours for the full effects. That way you can get a good gauge of how you feel and can adjust the dosage accordingly.

every body is different

Through experimentation and recipe testing for *Sous Weed*, we discovered that my mother's beginner dose is my maximum dose! That goes to show just how difficult it is to determine how each individual's body will absorb these cannabinoids. Age, gender, weight, inflammation levels, and even what you've eaten that day could factor into the variability of effects. I ended up taking a nice, long nap on the couch while mom felt energized enough to deep-clean the kitchen.

author's note

A low dose is my preference when it comes to gummies and candies; it means I can enjoy more than one piece at a time. For that reason, the recipes in this book are designed to be snackable—around 1 mg to 5 mg per piece, depending on the size of the candy mold used. For those who need a higher starting dosage, use more cannabis flower or a more potent strain when making your infusions.

note for all recipes

The yield and potency will change depending on the size of the mold and potency of the strain used in your infusion.

dosage estimation

It is impossible to properly estimate the THC or CBD content of your infusion without lab-tested cannabis or hemp material. Even so, there are many other variables that can affect the potency of your cannabis—from different strains to how the plant is grown to how it's processed and cured. The types of oils and fats used, heating methods, and temperature and time will also affect your infusion's end product.

To begin your home infusions, it's important to start with plant material that comes with a certificate of analysis (COA), an authenticated document that includes the phytocannabinoid measurements. To get a general dosage estimate, you can refer to the COA of your dry flower and do a bit of math. There are also at-home potency-testing devices on the market that you can purchase.

If you don't know the potency of your cannabis flower, you can make a general estimate by starting at 15 percent total phytocannabinoids.*

Flower weight (mg) 1 g = 1,000 mg	×	% Phytocannabinoids in flower	÷	Tbsp infusion liquid 2 cups = 32 tbsp	÷	Tsp 1 tbsp = 3 tsp
7,000 mg	×	0.15	÷	32	÷	3

10.9 mg per tsp

For the infusions in this cookbook, I used the strain Oregon Guava, which clocked in at 17.3 percent total phytocannabinoids in the COA.

Flower weight (mg) 1 g = 1,000 mg	×	% Phytocannabinoids in flower	÷	Tbsp infusion liquid 2 cups = 32 tbsp	÷	Tsp 1 tbsp = 3 tsp
7,000 mg	×	0.173	÷	32	÷	3

12.6 mg per tsp

* Please note, this calculation does not address the loss of phytocannabinoids due to various heating methods, evaporation, or use of certain oils, fats, and alcohol for infusion. Again, this is only a rough estimate of potency.

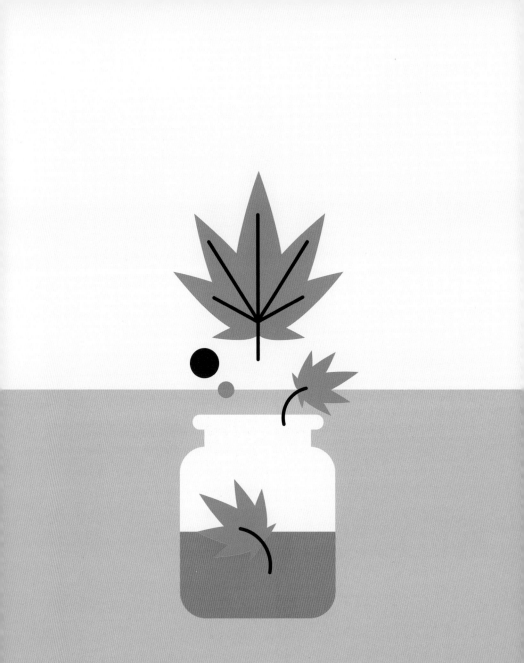

infusion basics

Before we begin candy making, a fully stocked pantry of cannabis infusions and sugars will help set your gummies up for success. Let's go back to the basics.

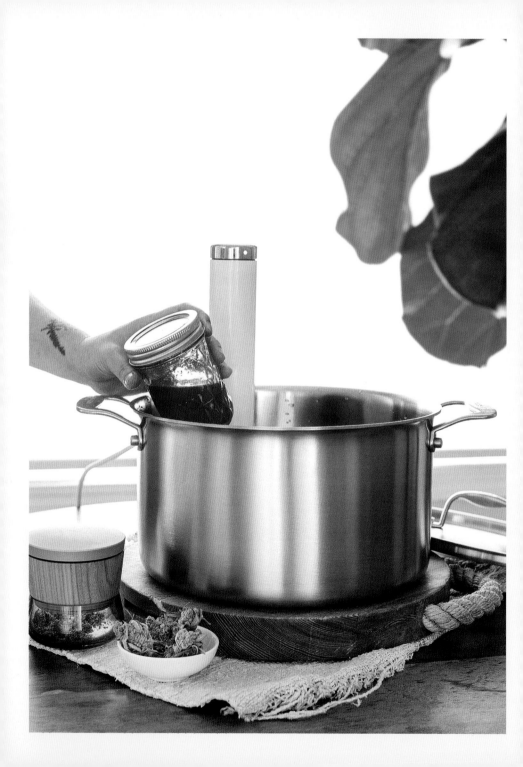

what is decarboxylation?

The first step to making your infusion is to activate the phytocanna-binoids in your cannabis with a process called decarboxylation. I promise it's not as complicated as it sounds, and there are various ways to do it. By decarboxylating your flower, you activate the THC and CBD in the cannabis or hemp to a higher potency before infusing it into your fat or alcohol base. For example, when heated, the phytocannabinoid tetrahydrocannabinolic acid (THCA) will convert to THC.

Activation Temperatures for Decarboxylation

Phytocannabinoids	Fahrenheit	Celsius
THCA	240°F–275°F	115°C–135°C
CBDA	240°F–295°F	115°C–146°C

THCA converts to THC when heated between 240°F and 275°F (115°C–135°C) for 20 minutes to 1 hour.

CBDA converts to CBD when heated between 240°F and 295°F (115°C–146°C) for 20 minutes to 1 hour.

Source: Jamie Evans, *The Ultimate Guide to CBD: Explore the World of Cannabidiol* (Beverley, MA: Fair Winds Press, 2020).

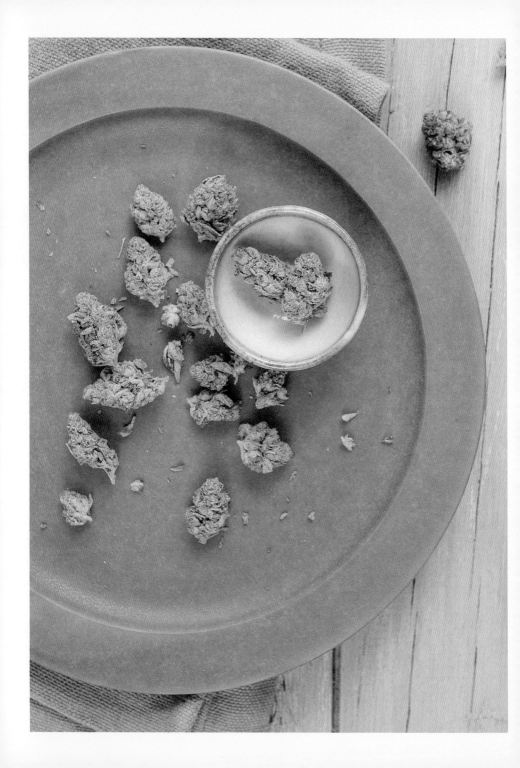

oven decarboxylation

Active Time
30 minutes

Ingredients
¼ ounce (7 g) cannabis flower

Author's Note
Kief, the loose, sticky dust that accumulates at the bottom of your herb grinder, can also be decarboxylated. Made up of dried trichomes, the tiny resin glands that cover the cannabis plant, it is more potent than cannabis flower so you can use less. Wrap the kief in a small foil packet before placing it in the oven to decarboxylate. We will use decarboxylated kief in the Kief-Infused Honey recipe (page 42).

I will be showing you my favorite method of decarboxylation (page 35), which requires a device called the Ardent FX, but you can always use your oven instead! Two things to note when using the oven method. One, oven temperatures tend to fluctuate at an average of 10 degrees so these temperatures are not always the most accurate. Two, it can be quite smelly so for those who would prefer discretion, I'd highly recommend looking into a sous vide machine or an Ardent FX.

1. Preheat the oven to 250°F (121°C) and line a sheet tray with parchment paper.

2. Break the cannabis flower into pea-size chunks and spread evenly on the sheet tray. Bake for 30 minutes.

3. Remove from the oven and use in your infusions.

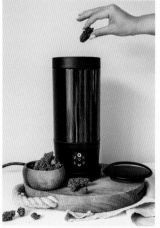 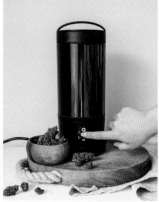 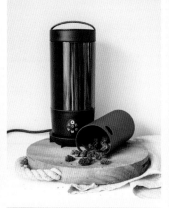
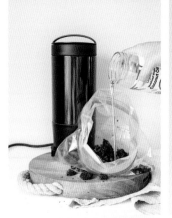 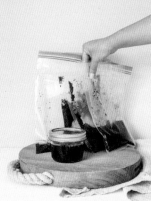 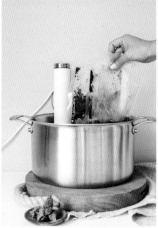
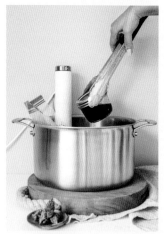 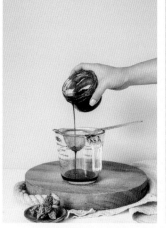 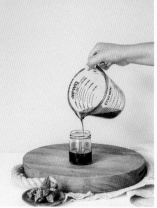

my at-home process: sous vide infusion

Active Time
varies

Ingredients
2 cups coconut or MCT oil
¼ ounce (7g) cannabis flower

Author's Note
The amount of flower specified in this recipe is a loose suggestion. Please refer to the dosage estimation chart (page 27) to calculate your dosage.

This is the exact workflow in my home kitchen. In terms of tools for this tutorial, I use the Ardent FX to effectively decarboxylate my flower and fully activate the THC and CBD with the touch of a button. While there are other ways to decarboxylate, this is my favorite method.

You will also need a sous vide machine for your infusions. Not only is it great for making multiple infusions at once, it's also useful for your daily cooking needs. After working on two sous vide cookbooks, I can confidently say that you will never again eat overcooked steak or chicken. It also makes the silkiest crème brûlée.

1. Use cannabis or hemp flower that's been lab tested for safety and potency. I used Oregon Guava, an incredibly aromatic CBD flower from Grow It From Home. You can use more or less flower depending on the desired potency of your oil.

2. To decarboxylate, place your whole cannabis flower in the Ardent FX and select A1 to activate the THC. If using hemp flower or a high CBD cannabis flower, select A2 to activate the CBD. With the decarboxylation process, the THC or CBD in the flower will activate to a higher potency before you infuse it into your oil base.

3. The decarboxylated flower should smell nutty and toasty. Now it's ready to be used in your oil infusion. Place the flower into a quart-size freezer-safe ziplock bag, vacuum-seal bag, silicone sous vide bag, or even a mason jar.*

4. Add in the oil of your choice and be sure to push the air out of the bag before sealing. This will ensure the bag stays submerged underwater. (One of the best parts of the sous vide method is being able to make multiple infusions at once! Here I

my at-home process
continued

have coconut oil, olive oil, butter, avocado oil, and sesame oil about to go into a water bath.)

5. Set your sous vide water bath to 185°F (85°C). Once the sous vide water bath has reached its temperature, submerge the sealed bags or jars in the water bath. Sous vide for 4 hours.

6. After the oil has finished infusing, gently remove the jars or bags from the water bath, using tongs.

7. Using a fine-mesh strainer or cheesecloth, strain out the solids and discard the spent flower. Store infused oils, such as sesame, avocado, coconut, and olive oil, in airtight jars in a cool, dark place. Infused butter, lard, or other animal fats should be stored in the fridge.

*When using a mason jar, there are several safety rules to follow to prevent the glass from breaking in the water bath. Always inspect the jars for any cracks or scratches before use. Screw the jar lids only "finger tight." Applying too much pressure to the screw band will cause the jar to crack in the water bath. Mason jars should be placed in the water early, as it's starting to heat up, to prevent thermal shock.

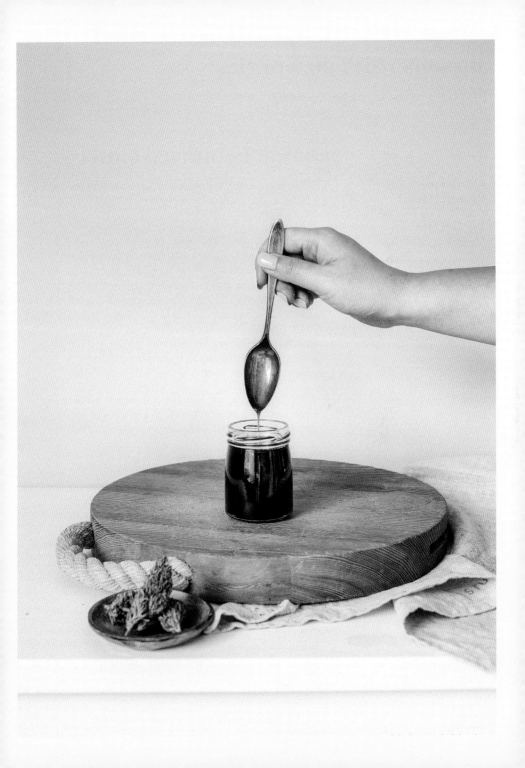

no sous vide? no worries!

Next up are some recipes for basic cannabis infusions that can be made without a special sous vide device.

cannabis-infused butter

Active Time
3½ hours

Inactive Time
12 hours

Ingredients
2 cups unsalted butter, melted
2 cups water
¼ ounce (7 g) cannabis flower, decarboxylated

Author's Note
Most store-bought butter has 15%–20% water content, which will be lost in the end product. Make sure to begin with melted butter and make sure it yields 2 cups before starting the infusion process.

1. Place the melted butter, water, and decarboxylated cannabis flower in a large mason jar. Seal the jar finger tight.

2. Set the mason jar in a medium saucepan and fill the saucepan with water, making sure it does not reach the top of the mason jar. Set the heat to medium low and clip a candy thermometer to the saucepan. Bring to a simmer and keep the temperature around 200°F (93°C), never exceeding 211°F (99°C). Cook for 3 hours, checking in often to refill the saucepan with water as needed. Once every hour, gently shake the mason jar while wearing an oven mitt.

3. After 3 hours, gently remove the mason jar with an oven mitt and allow the infusion to cool to room temperature, about an hour.

4. Prepare a cheesecloth and set it over a fine-mesh strainer. Pour the cannabis-infused butter mixture through the cheesecloth and into a measuring cup with a spout. Do not wring the cheesecloth, the leftover plant material may leave an acrid taste. Discard the solids. Transfer the butter mixture to the fridge overnight to solidify and separate from the water.

5. Remove the butter from the fridge. Using a knife, loosen the sides of the cannabis-infused butter and transfer the block to a clean container. Discard the water. Store the infused butter in the fridge.

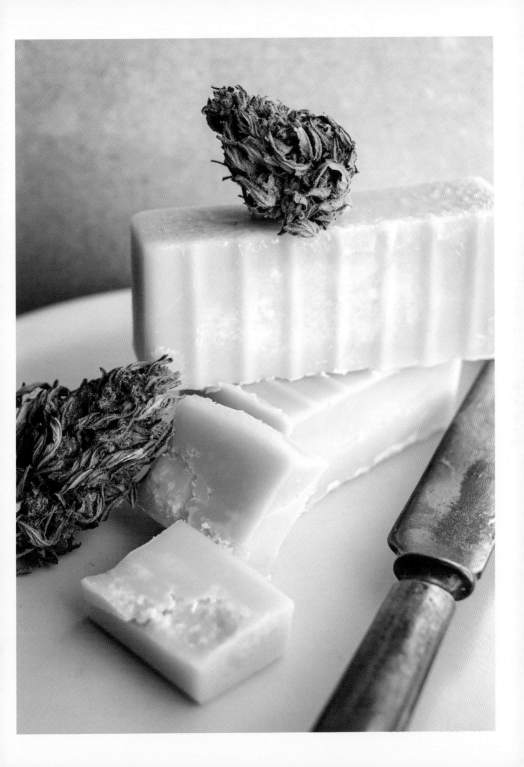

cannabis-infused MCT oil

Active Time
2½ hours

Inactive Time
1 hour

Ingredients
2 cups MCT oil or
coconut oil
¼ ounce (7 g) cannabis
flower, decarboxylated

1. Place coconut or MCT oil along with decarboxylated cannabis flower in a mason jar. Seal the top finger tight.

2. Set the mason jar in a medium saucepan and fill the saucepan with water, making sure it does not reach the top of the mason jar. Set the heat to medium-low and clip a candy thermometer to the saucepan. Bring to a simmer and keep the temperature around 200°F (93°C), never exceeding 211°F (99°C). Cook for 2 hours, checking in often to refill the saucepan with water as needed. Once every hour, gently shake the mason jar while wearing an oven mitt.

3. After 2 hours, gently remove the mason jar with an oven mitt and allow the infusion to cool to room temperature, about an hour.

4. Prepare a cheesecloth and set it over a fine-mesh strainer. Pour the cannabis-infused MCT oil through the cheesecloth and into a measuring cup with a spout. Do not wring the cheesecloth—the leftover plant material may leave an acrid taste. Discard the solids. Transfer the finished oil to clean jars or tincture bottles. Store in a cool, dark place.

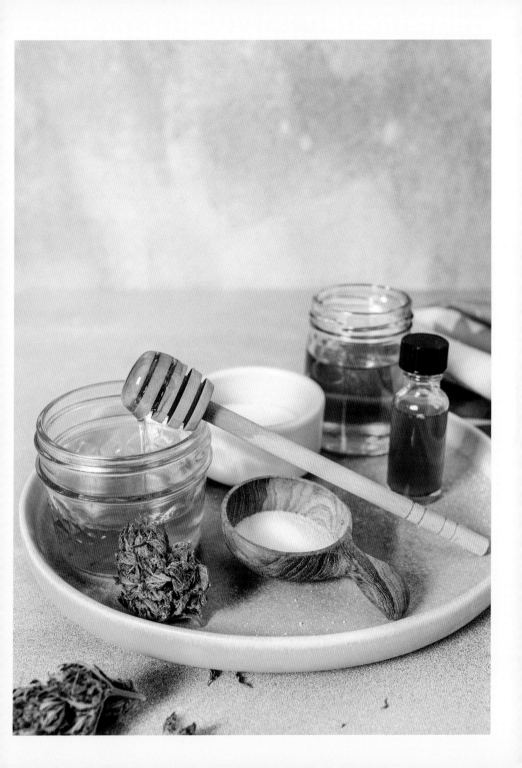

kief-infused honey

Active Time
1 hour

Ingredients
2 cups honey
2g kief, decarboxylated
(page 33)

1. Add 2 inches of water to the bottom pan of your double boiler* and set the heat to medium low. Once the water comes to a boil, set the top double boiler pan or bowl on the bottom pan and add the honey and decarboxylated kief.

2. Cook for 1 hour, checking it often to refill the bottom pan with water as needed. Stir occasionally.

3. After an hour, transfer the infused honey to a clean jar (there is no need to strain out the kief). Store the honey in a cool, dark place. Stir well before use.

You can also sous vide the kief-infused honey for ease.

cannabis-infused tincture

Active Time
5 minutes

Inactive Time
24 hours

___

Ingredients

¼ ounce (7 g) cannabis flower, decarboxylated

2 cups high-proof alcohol, like Everclear or a strong grain alcohol

A massive thank you to Ardent for sharing this Cannabis-Infused Tincture recipe along with the lab test results, which can be found on their website, ardentcannabis.com.

1. Place the decarboxylated cannabis flower inside an empty mason jar and pour the grain alcohol over the top, covering the flower completely. Close the mason jar securely.

2. Store the jar in a cool, dark place such as a cupboard or closet, giving it a good shake every few hours to agitate the alcohol infusion. It will be ready to use within 24 hours.*

3. Prepare a cheesecloth and set it over a fine-mesh strainer. Pour the cannabis-infused tincture through the cheesecloth and into a measuring cup with a spout. Discard the solids. Transfer the finished tincture to clean jars or bottles. Store in a cool, dark place.

Ardent's lab testing shows that with a 3-hour Everclear soak, there is already significant cannabinoid extraction of over 80 percent. If you can wait longer, the additional overnight soak will give full potency.

cannabis-infused sugar

By taking Ardent's Cannabis-Infused Tincture process (page 43) one step further, you can make a simple Cannabis-Infused Sugar.

Active Time
5 minutes

Inactive Time
24 hours

Ingredients

1 cup granulated sugar

¼ cup Cannabis-Infused Tincture (page 43)

1. Spread out the sugar on a baking sheet lined with parchment paper. Pour the cannabis tincture over the sugar and mix it around. Leave the tray out in the open for the alcohol to evaporate. Stir every few hours and make tracks in the sugar to assist with airflow.

2. After 24 hours, the cannabis-infused sugar should look light gold in color. If the dried sugar is clumped together, gently break apart the larger chunks with the back of a large wooden spoon.

3. Store the cannabis-infused sugar in an airtight container.

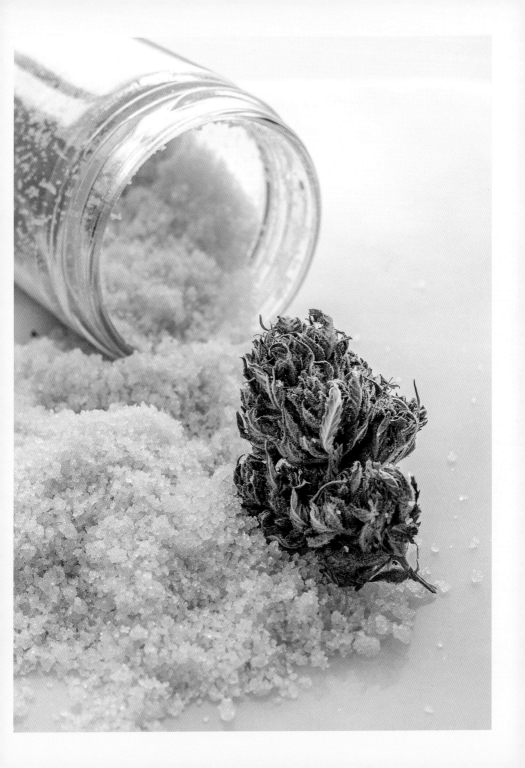

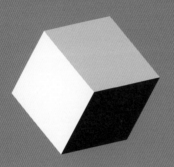
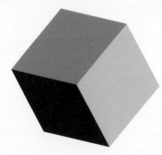

1

gummies & jellies

The gummies in this chapter are made of a combination of sweeteners, gelling agents, a cannabis infusion, and natural flavorings.

Since these gummies are made primarily with natural ingredients, they will have a shorter shelf life at room temperature than store-bought gummies that are laden with preservatives. But fret not! They will last longer in the fridge or freezer.

note for all recipes

The yield and potency will change depending on the size of the mold and potency of the strain used in your infusion.

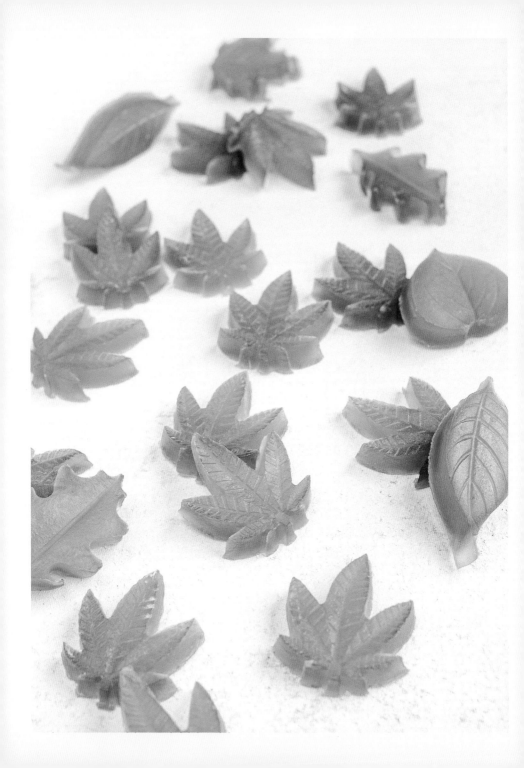

sour green apple gummies

Active Time
15 minutes

Inactive Time
2 to 12 hours

Ingredients

¼ cup cold water

¼ cup grass-fed gelatin powder

¾ cup green apple juice, fresh

2 tablespoons granulated sugar

¼ cup light corn syrup

1 tablespoon Cannabis-Infused MCT Oil (page 40)

½ teaspoon sunflower lecithin

½ teaspoon citric acid

green food coloring (optional)

¼ cup plus 2 tablespoons cornstarch, divided (optional)

2 tablespoons powdered sugar (optional)

We're starting with a classic sour green apple gummy made with fresh green apple juice. Some of the ingredients may look unfamiliar, so let's break it down. The sunflower lecithin will help bind the water, apple juice, and cannabis-infused MCT oil together. The citric acid adds that sour punch that we all expect in a green apple flavor. Finally, the addition of light corn syrup and the dusting of cornstarch help give the gummies a more distinctive, commercial texture.

1. Pour the cold water into a small bowl and sprinkle the grass-fed gelatin powder over the surface. Whisk with a fork to combine and allow to bloom for 5 minutes.

2. In a small saucepan over medium heat, bring the green apple juice, granulated sugar, and light corn syrup to a boil. Remove from the heat and add the cannabis-infused MCT oil, sunflower lecithin, citric acid, and 2 to 3 drops of food coloring, if using. Whisk to fully combine the ingredients.

3. Add in the bloomed gelatin and gently stir until the gelatin has completely melted and the mixture is uniform. Use a measuring cup with a spout or a candy dropper to fill your gummy mold. Chill in the fridge until firm, 1 to 2 hours.* Gently remove the gummies from the mold and enjoy.

Curing Your Gummies

1. For a firmer texture, cure the gummies by transferring them to a wire rack for 12 hours at room temperature or uncovered in the fridge if the room is too humid. If there is too much humidity, toss the gummies in a ¼ cup of the cornstarch, if using, before placing on the wire rack. After the cure, dust off any excess cornstarch with a pastry brush or rinse off the cornstarch with cold water and allow the gummies to air-dry.

sour green apple gummies
continued

2. To coat your gummies with a little extra sweetness, mix the remaining 2 tablespoons of cornstarch and the powdered sugar, if using, in a bowl. Toss the gummies in this mixture until evenly coated and brush off any excess. The cornstarch will also keep the gummies from sticking to each other.

3. Store in a cool, dry room-temperature location for up to 5 days. Gummies will last up to 2 weeks in the fridge when stored in an airtight container. Gummies can also be stored in the freezer for up to 6 months.

* If it's difficult to unmold your gummies, freeze them for an hour to make them easier to pop out.

lavender chamomile sleep gummies

Active Time
25 minutes

Inactive Time
2 to 12 hours

Ingredients
¼ cup cold water, plus 1 cup water for tea

¼ cup grass-fed gelatin powder

2 teaspoons dried chamomile

2 teaspoons dried lavender

2 teaspoons fresh mint, chopped

3 tablespoons granulated sugar

¼ cup honey

1 tablespoon Cannabis-Infused MCT Oil (page 40)

½ teaspoon sunflower lecithin

purple food coloring (optional)

Author's Note
Refer back to the cornstarch curing method (page 49) if you live in a humid region or if your gummies need additional firming up.

Whether it's thinking about work or if our chihuahua's favorite parent is me or David, it's sometimes hard to unwind at night. I like to have a mug of soothing chamomile and lavender tea or a gummy with the same flavor to help me sleep. If you have a particular cannabis strain that you prefer to consume in the evening, this is the perfect opportunity to infuse it into MCT oil or a tincture to use in this gummy.

1. Pour the ¼ cup of cold water into a small bowl and sprinkle the grass-fed gelatin powder over the surface. Whisk with a fork to combine and allow to bloom for 5 minutes.

2. Make tea: Bring the remaining water to a boil in a small saucepan and then remove from heat. Add the chamomile, lavender, mint, granulated sugar, and honey; stir to combine. Steep for 15 minutes.

3. Strain out the solids and discard. Bring the mixture back to a boil on medium heat for 3 minutes. Remove from the heat and add the cannabis-infused MCT oil, sunflower lecithin, and 2 to 3 drops of food coloring, if using. Whisk to fully combine the ingredients.

4. Add in the bloomed gelatin and gently stir until the gelatin has completely melted and the mixture is uniform. Use a measuring cup with a spout or a candy dropper to fill your gummy mold.

5. Chill in the fridge until firm, 1 to 2 hours. Gently remove the gummies from the mold and enjoy.

6. Store in a cool, dry room-temperature location for up to 5 days. Gummies will last up to 2 weeks in the fridge when stored in an airtight container. Gummies can also be stored in the freezer for up to 6 months.

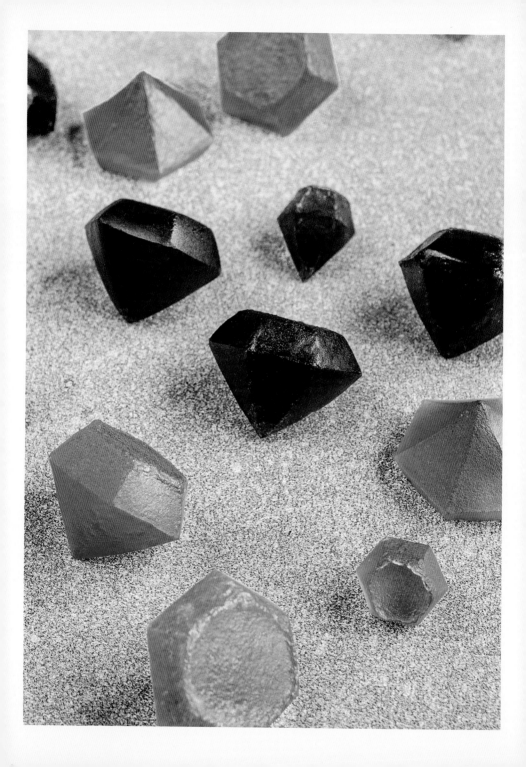

sour pink lemonade gummies

Active Time
15 minutes

Inactive Time
2 to 12 hours

Ingredients

¼ cup cold water

¼ cup grass-fed gelatin powder

½ cup cranberry juice

3 tablespoons granulated sugar

¼ cup light corn syrup

¼ cup lemon juice, fresh

1 tablespoon Cannabis-Infused MCT Oil (page 40)

½ teaspoon sunflower lecithin

½ teaspoon citric acid

pink food coloring (optional)

Author's Note
Refer back to the cornstarch curing method (page 49) if you live in a humid region or if your gummies need additional firming up.

This gummy is an ode to my inner '90s kid. It's a throwback to special occasions at the local pizza buffet and chugging copious amounts of pink lemonade; normally I was never allowed this much sugar during mealtime. In this recipe, the pink color comes from cranberry juice, which also adds a nice balance of sweet and tart. Depending on the intensity of pink you're looking for, 1 or 2 drops of pink food coloring in the mixture will really make the gummies pop.

1. Pour the cold water into a small bowl and sprinkle the grass-fed gelatin powder over the surface. Whisk with a fork to combine and allow to bloom for 5 minutes.

2. In a small saucepan over medium heat, bring the cranberry juice, granulated sugar, and light corn syrup to a boil. Remove from the heat and add the lemon juice, cannabis-infused MCT oil, sunflower lecithin, citric acid, and 2 to 3 drops of the optional food coloring. Whisk to fully combine the ingredients.

3. Add in the bloomed gelatin and gently stir until the gelatin has completely melted and the mixture is uniform. Use a measuring cup with a spout or a candy dropper to fill your gummy mold.

4. Chill in the fridge until firm, 1 to 2 hours. Gently remove the gummies from the mold and enjoy.

5. Store in a cool, dry room-temperature location for up to 5 days. Gummies will last up to 2 weeks in the fridge when stored in an airtight container. Gummies can also be stored in the freezer for up to 6 months.

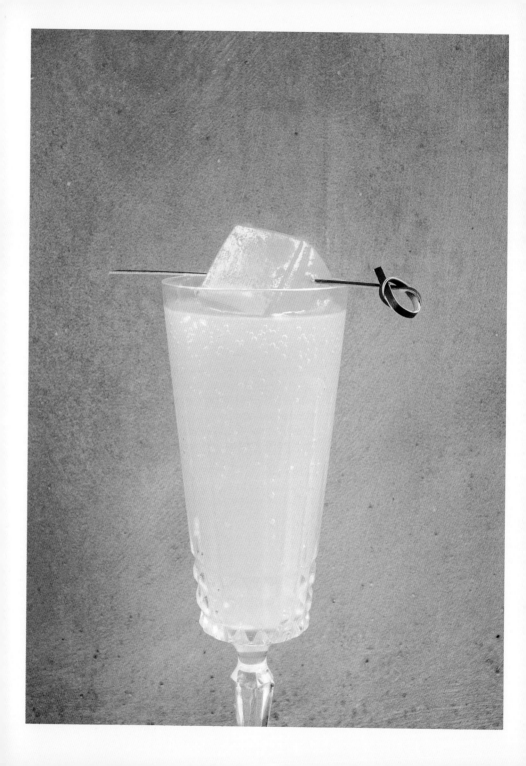

mimosa gummies

This recipe is born out of my love for day drinking. Make these mimosa gummies with your favorite sparkling wine, or, if you're "California sober," a nonalcoholic sparkling wine will taste just as lovely. For a mold, I used a silicone ice cube tray and served the gummy as a garnish in a mimosa during brunch.

Active Time

15 minutes

Inactive Time

2 to 12 hours

Ingredients

¼ cup cold water

¼ cup grass-fed gelatin powder

½ cup orange juice

½ cup prosecco, cava, or nonalcoholic sparkling wine

3 tablespoons granulated sugar

¼ cup light corn syrup

1 tablespoon Cannabis-Infused Tincture (page 43)

½ teaspoon citric acid

Author's Note

Refer back to the cornstarch curing method (page 49) if you live in a humid region or if your gummies need additional firming up.

1. Pour the cold water into a small bowl and sprinkle the grass-fed gelatin powder over the surface. Whisk with a fork to combine and allow to bloom for 5 minutes.

2. In a small saucepan over medium heat, bring the orange juice, sparkling wine, granulated sugar, and light corn syrup to a boil for 3 minutes. Remove from the heat and add the cannabis-infused tincture and citric acid. Whisk to fully combine the ingredients.

3. Add in the bloomed gelatin and gently stir until the gelatin has completely melted and the mixture is uniform. Use a measuring cup with a spout or a candy dropper to fill your gummy mold.

4. Chill in the fridge until firm, 1 to 2 hours. Gently remove the gummies from the mold and enjoy.

5. Store in a cool, dry room-temperature location for up to 5 days. Gummies will last up to 2 weeks in the fridge when stored in an airtight container. Gummies can also be stored in the freezer for up to 6 months.

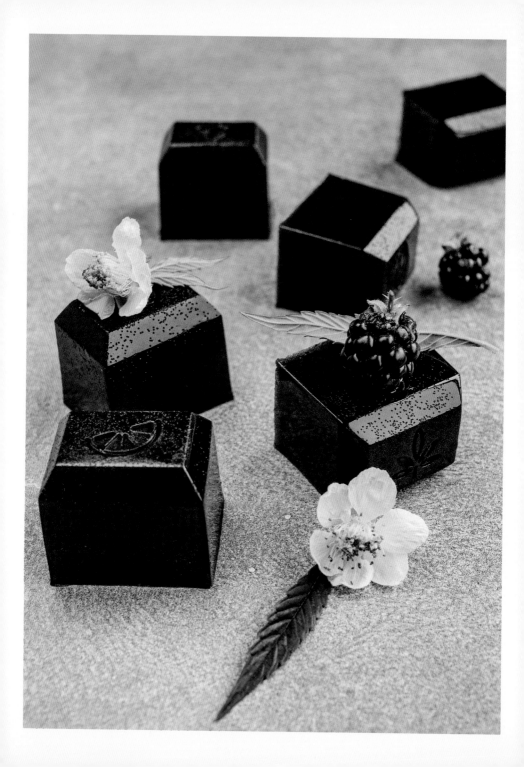

blackberry thyme gummies

Active Time
20 minutes

Inactive Time
2 to 12 hours

Ingredients

½ cup blackberries, fresh or defrosted

juice of ½ lemon

¼ cup cold water, plus ¾ cup water for tea

¼ cup grass-fed gelatin powder

1 black tea bag

2 sprigs thyme

¼ cup honey

3 tablespoons granulated sugar

1 tablespoon Cannabis-Infused Tincture (page 43)

Author's Note
Refer back to the cornstarch curing method (page 49) if you live in a humid region or if your gummies need additional firming up.

A thorny blackberry bush has aggressively taken over our fence this summer. I'm not complaining, though; we've picked fat, juicy berries to enjoy every day. This blackberry thyme gummy is inspired by the fruits and herbs in my garden. We put a lot of hard labor and love into this year's harvest, which is why I adore this recipe.

1. Puree the blackberries and lemon juice in a food processor and strain out the seeds using a fine-mesh strainer. Set the blackberry juice aside.

2. Pour ¼ cup cold water into a small bowl and sprinkle the grass-fed gelatin powder over the surface. Whisk with a fork to combine and allow to bloom for 5 minutes.

3. Make tea: Bring ¾ cup water to a boil in a small saucepan and remove from the heat. Add the black tea bag, thyme, and honey. Stir to combine and steep for 5 minutes.

4. Strain out the tea bag and solids and discard. Add the blackberry juice and granulated sugar to the tea and stir to combine. Bring the mixture to a light boil for 3 minutes. Remove from the heat, add the cannabis-infused tincture, and whisk to combine the ingredients.

5. Add in the bloomed gelatin and gently stir until the gelatin has completely melted and the mixture is uniform. Remove any bubbles that may have formed. Use a measuring cup with a spout or a candy dropper to fill your gummy mold.

6. Chill in the fridge until firm, 1 to 2 hours. Gently remove the gummies from the mold and enjoy.

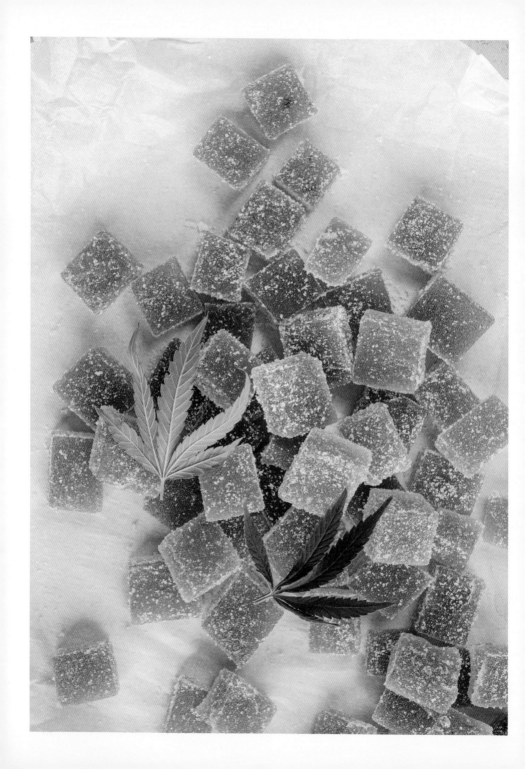

spiced orange
pâte de fruit

Makes 64 squares

Active Time
30 minutes

Inactive Time
24 hours

Ingredients

4¼ cups granulated sugar, divided*

2⅓ tablespoons rapid-set HM pectin

2 cups orange juice

zest of 1 orange

¼ cup lemon juice

2 cinnamon sticks

1 teaspoon whole cloves

¼ cup Kief-Infused Honey (page 42)

1 teaspoon citric acid

Special Equipment

large heavy-bottomed saucepan

candy or instant-read thermometer

8-inch square baking pan

Nothing gets me in the mood for the holidays like the smell of orange zest and warming spices. This orange pomander-inspired pâte de fruit is one of my favorite recipes in this book and a crowd favorite. These little candy gems look so sophisticated packaged up for gift giving or presented on the dessert table.

1. Line an 8-inch square baking pan with a sheet of parchment paper. Crease the corners along the inside edges and leave a 1-inch overhang on each side of the pan.

2. In a small bowl, combine ¼ cup of sugar and the rapid-set HM pectin.

3. In a large heavy-bottomed saucepan, whisk together the orange juice, orange zest, lemon juice, cinnamon sticks, and cloves. Set over medium-high heat and bring to a boil for 15 minutes to infuse spices. Scoop out the cinnamon sticks and cloves and discard. Whisk in the kief-infused honey and sugar-pectin mixture and lower the heat to medium low.

4. Whisk in 1½ cups of sugar and continue whisking until the mixture returns to a boil. Add another 1½ cups of sugar and continue to whisk until the mixture returns to a boil. Clip a candy thermometer to the saucepan. Continue cooking the mixture until it reaches 225°F (107°C), whisking constantly to prevent burning.

5. Remove from the heat and stir in the citric acid; beware of steam as you stir. Evenly pour the hot pâte de fruit mixture into the prepared 8-inch square baking pan. Cool to room temperature, about 2 hours.

spiced orange pâte de fruit

continued

6. Gently release the pâte de fruit from the baking pan by lifting the parchment paper and set on a work surface. Sprinkle granulated sugar on both sides of the pâte de fruit to make it easier to handle.

7. Using a sharp knife, cut the pâte de fruit into 1-inch squares and toss the squares in the remaining granulated sugar until all sides are coated.

8. Enjoy now or take the extra step to cure the pâte de fruit by placing the squares on a baking sheet lined with parchment paper. Allow the pâte de fruit to cure, uncovered, at room temperature for 24 hours to create a crisp sugar crust. Store in an airtight container with a desiccant packet for up to a month.

* For a more potent pâte de fruit, substitute the 1 cup of granulated sugar used for coating with homemade cannabis-infused sugar.

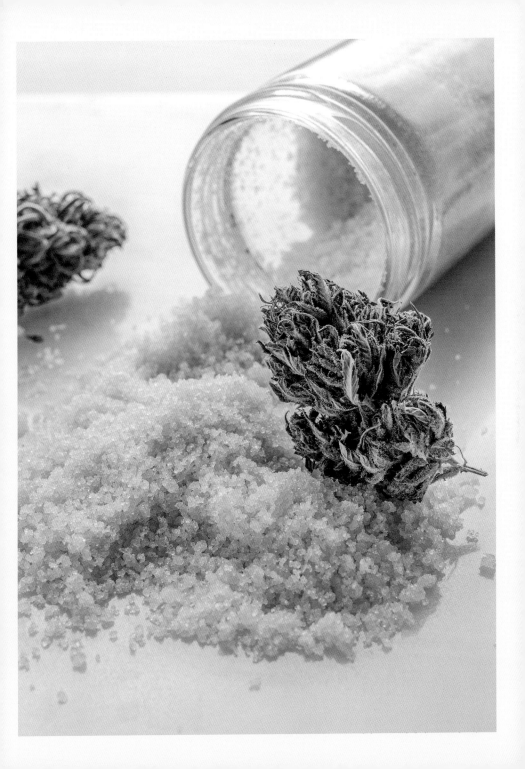

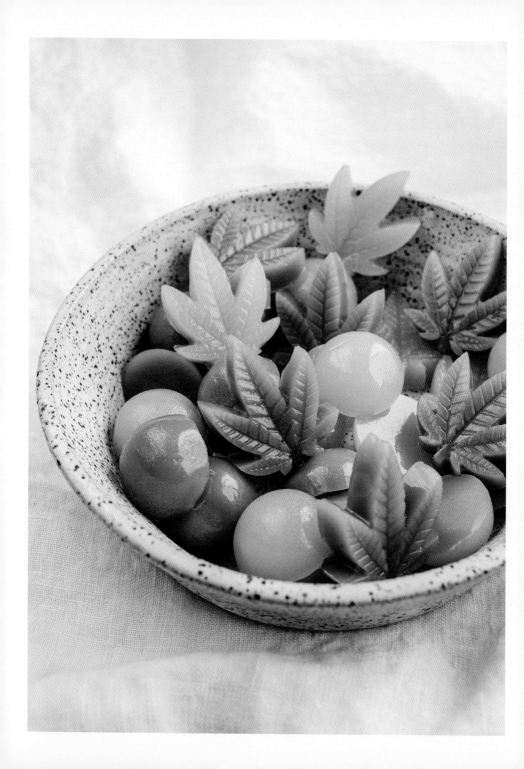

kombucha gummies

Active Time
15 minutes

Inactive Time
30 minutes

Ingredients

¼ cup water

2 teaspoons agar-agar powder

2 tablespoons granulated sugar

¼ cup Kief-Infused Honey (page 42)

1 cup kombucha of your choice

¼ teaspoon citric acid

Kombucha is a fermented, probiotic-rich wellness beverage that dates back to ancient China. If you're down with the funk, the use of kombucha makes for a unique and tangy gummy. The flavor will change based on the type of kombucha you select, so play around with a few different brands, or brew your own if you're feeling crafty!

1. Add the water, agar-agar powder, and granulated sugar to a small saucepan and whisk the mixture together.

2. Add in the kief-infused honey and kombucha and turn up the heat to medium. Bring the mixture to a gentle simmer for 3 minutes to activate the agar-agar. Stir often to completely melt the agar-agar powder. Remove from the heat and add the citric acid. Stir until the mixture is completely uniform.

3. Use a measuring cup with a spout or a candy dropper to fill your gummy mold.

4. Chill in the fridge until firm, 20 to 30 minutes. Pop the gummies out of the mold and enjoy.

5. Store in an airtight container in the fridge.

green juice gummies

Active Time
15 minutes

Inactive Time
30 minutes

Ingredients

¼ cup water

2 teaspoons agar-agar powder

2 tablespoons granulated sugar

¼ cup Kief-Infused Honey (page 42)

1 cup green juice of your choice

¼ teaspoon citric acid

Author's Note

Is cannabis the new kale? I love juicing the nutrient-dense leaves of my cannabis and hemp plants. It is especially delicious mixed with ginger and pineapple juice.

We all know about the wonderful health benefits of a daily glass of green juice. Unfortunately, my juicer sits unused most of the time because it is far too labor intensive to prep produce every single morning. Green juice in gummy form is something I can get behind, though. Make a large batch for the week using a CBD-heavy strain to help get your day started off right. Use a green juice of your choice and include some fruit juice, such as apple or pineapple, to add extra sweetness to the gummy.

1. Add the water, agar-agar powder, and granulated sugar to a small saucepan and whisk the mixture together.

2. Add in the kief-infused honey and green juice and turn up the heat to medium. Bring the mixture to a gentle simmer for 3 minutes to activate the agar-agar. Stir often to completely melt the agar-agar powder. Remove from the heat and add the citric acid. Stir until the mixture is completely uniform.

3. Use a measuring cup with a spout or a candy dropper to fill your gummy mold.

4. Chill in the fridge until firm, 20 to 30 minutes. Pop the gummies out of the mold and enjoy.

5. Store in an airtight container in the fridge.

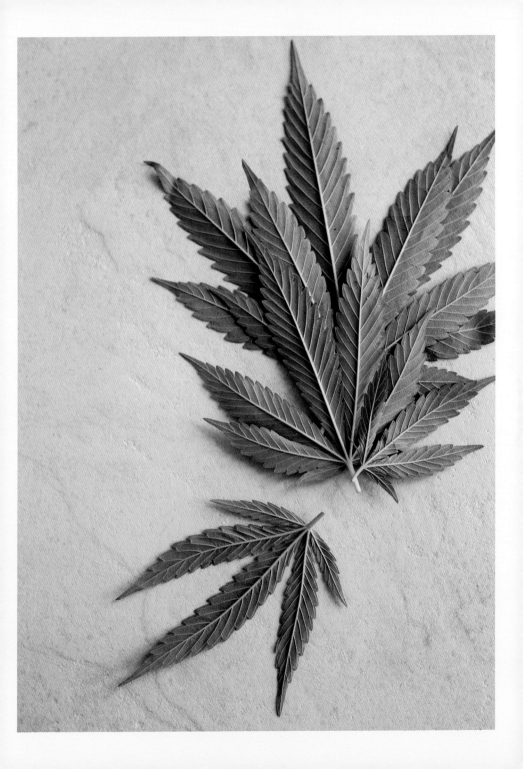

terrazzo coffee jelly

Makes 8 servings

Active Time
35 minutes

Inactive Time
1 hour

Ingredients for Coffee Jelly

2 teaspoons agar-agar powder

2 cups brewed coffee, cold

1 tablespoon granulated sugar

Ingredients for Coconut Milk Jelly

½ cup water

4 teaspoons agar-agar powder

¼ cup granulated sugar

2 (13.5-ounce) cans unsweetened coconut milk

2 tablespoons Cannabis-Infused Sugar (page 44)

½ teaspoon vanilla extract

Special Equipment
8-inch square baking pan

This dessert is one I remember my mom making for brunch parties with her friends. Her version was more meticulous, with thin alternating layers of coffee and coconut cream jelly, but this quicker method looks striking as well. The wonderful thing about agar-agar is that it remains stable even in warm weather, meaning these sweet treats are excellent for picnics or potlucks where there's no refrigeration.

1. To make the coffee jelly, add the agar-agar powder, cold coffee, and granulated sugar to a small saucepan and whisk to combine, making sure there are no clumps.

2. Turn up the heat to medium and bring the mixture to a boil for 5 minutes to activate the agar-agar powder, stirring often. Pour into an 8-inch square baking pan. Refrigerate until solid, about 15 minutes.

3. Remove the coffee jelly from the fridge and unmold. Cut into cubes of varying sizes and scatter inside the 8-inch square baking pan. Set aside.

4. To make the coconut milk jelly, add the water, agar-agar powder, and granulated sugar to a medium saucepan and whisk to combine, making sure there are no clumps.

5. Add the coconut milk to the saucepan, turn the heat to medium, and bring the mixture to a boil for 5 minutes to activate the agar-agar, stirring often. Remove from the heat and add in the cannabis-infused sugar and vanilla extract. Stir until the sugar has fully dissolved. Pour into the 8-inch square baking pan with the coffee jelly. Refrigerate until solid, about an hour.

6. Cut into 2 x 4-inch rectangles to serve. Store in the fridge.

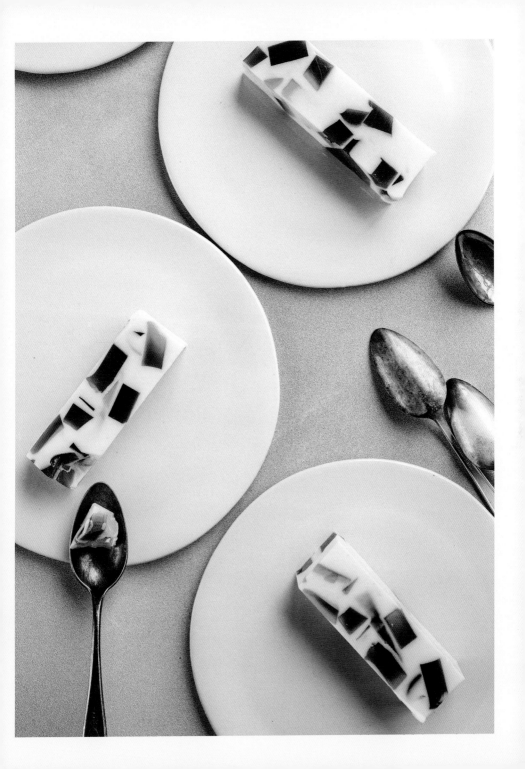

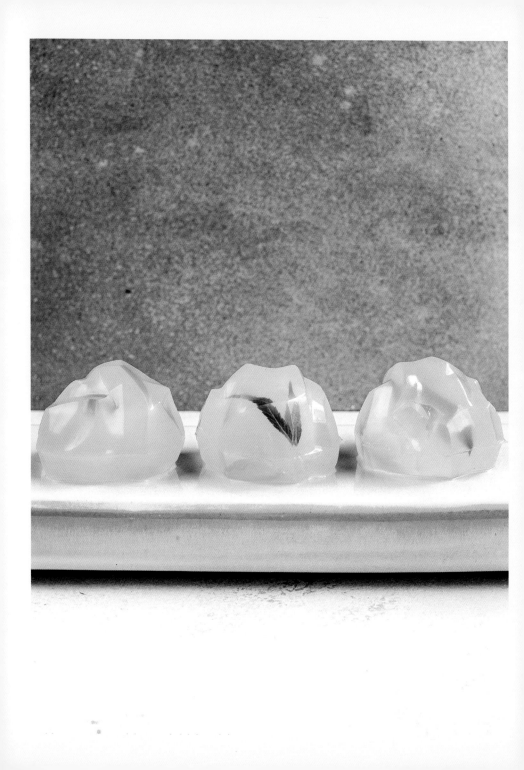

lychee jelly

Makes 3 (2½-inch) jellies

Active Time
10 minutes

Inactive Time
30 minutes

Ingredients

1½ teaspoons agar-agar

1 cup lychee syrup, strained from 1 (20-ounce) can lychees in heavy syrup, plus 3 lychees

2 teaspoons Cannabis-Infused Sugar (page 44)

3 small cannabis leaves (optional)

edible flowers (optional)

Special Equipment

3 (2½-inch) spherical ice cube mold

Inspired by the trendy raindrop jelly cake, this treat is made with lychee, edible flowers, and tiny cannabis sugar leaves. It's sure to impress guests at your next dinner party.

1. Add the agar-agar powder and lychee syrup to a small saucepan and whisk to combine.

2. Turn up the heat to medium and bring the mixture to a boil for 3 minutes to activate the agar-agar, stirring often. Remove from the heat and add in the cannabis-infused sugar. Stir until the sugar has fully dissolved. Pour into a measuring cup with a spout.

3. Add a lychee and any floral and leaf garnishes, if using, to each spherical ice cube mold. Gently fill the molds with the mixture.

4. Chill in the fridge until firm, 20 to 30 minutes. Pop the jellies from the molds and enjoy. Store in the fridge.

gemstone gummies

Makes 32 pieces

Active Time
1½ hours

Inactive Time
2 to 4 days

Ingredients

3 cups granulated sugar

6 teaspoons agar-agar powder

2 cups cold water

¼ cup Cannabis-Infused Sugar (page 44)

½ teaspoon super-strength candy flavoring of your choice

food coloring of your choice

Special Equipment

8-inch square baking pan

fine-mesh strainer

toothpicks

disposable gloves

When I moved to San Francisco, I had the privilege of living within walking distance of Japantown. After work, I would peruse the candy and snack aisles of the grocery stores and pop my head into various confectionery shops. This gummy is based on the traditional Japanese rock candy called kohakutou. It's a stunning-looking treat with a crunchy, crystalized exterior and a gummy center. The fun part of this recipe is swirling together your favorite colors to create an arresting gemstone appearance. I've used a touch of green, yellow, and white to create a jade-like effect.

1. Line an 8-inch square baking pan with a sheet of parchment paper. Crease the corners along the inside edges and leave a 1-inch overhang on each side of the pan. Lightly coat with nonstick spray.

2. Add the sugar, agar-agar powder, and water to a medium heavy-bottomed saucepan and stir with a silicone spatula to combine.

3. Turn the heat to medium and bring to a boil. Lower the heat and simmer for 8 minutes to activate the agar-agar and thicken the mixture, stirring often. Remove from the heat and add the cannabis-infused sugar and your candy flavoring of choice, stirring until the sugar has dissolved into the mixture.

4. Pour the mixture through a fine-mesh strainer into the prepared baking pan. Using toothpicks dipped in food coloring, make colorful swirls in the mixture while still warm. Transfer to the fridge to cool until firm, 1 to 2 hours.

5. Remove from the pan by pulling on the parchment paper. Slice the slab into eight 1-inch strips. Wearing disposable gloves, roughly rip the gummies into 1 x 2-inch pieces and place onto a parchment paper-lined baking sheet.

6. Allow to dry in the open air at room temperature for 2 to 4 days, rotating sides each day, until a hard sugar crust has crystallized on the exterior. Store in an airtight container or candy bags for up to a month.

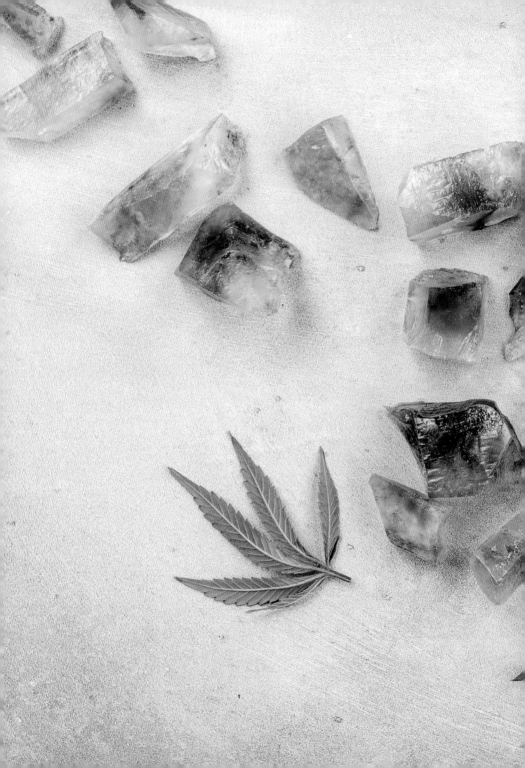

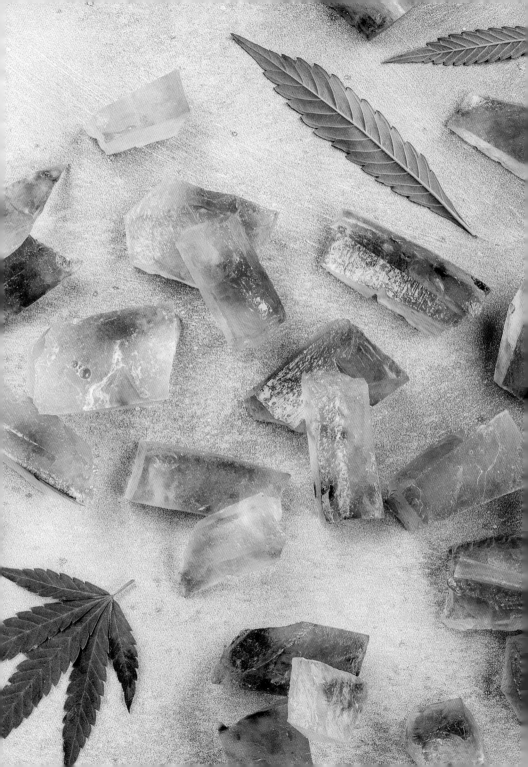

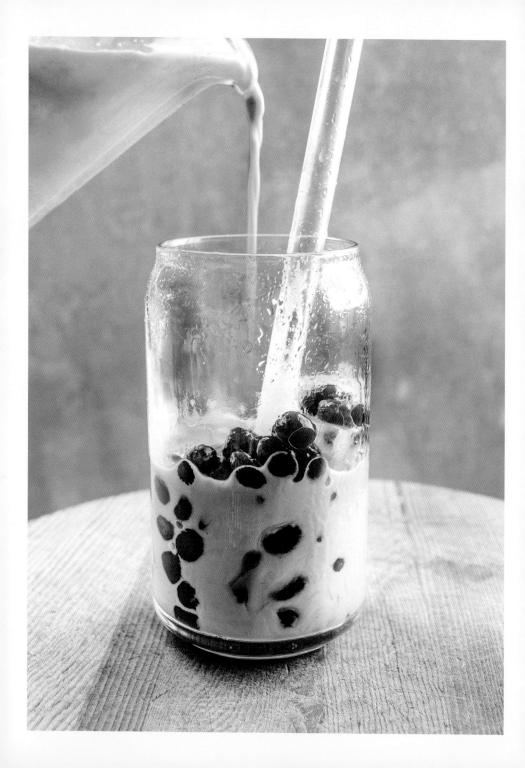

'bubble tea

Makes 4 servings

Active Time
1½ hours

Inactive Time
1 hour

Ingredients

¼ cup water

⅓ cup plus 1 tablespoon dark brown sugar, divided

1 tablespoon molasses

¾ cup tapioca flour, plus more for dusting

2 teaspoons Kief-Infused Honey (page 42)

¼ cup hot water

Special Equipment

baking sheet

medium heavy-bottomed saucepan

dough scraper

fine-mesh strainer

Oftentimes premade, store-bought tapioca balls are chock-full of preservatives and unhealthy additives to extend their shelf life. Making tapioca balls from scratch is tedious and time-consuming, but it can also be a fun project if you put your friends or family to work with you. The warm, robust flavor of molasses in the tapioca dough adds an extra-flavorful kick to your bubble tea (a.k.a. boba) creation.

1. Add ¼ cup water, 1 tablespoon of the dark brown sugar, and the molasses to a medium heavy-bottomed saucepan set over medium heat. Bring to a boil, stirring with a silicone spatula until the sugar has dissolved.

2. Turn the heat off and add 1 tablespoon of the tapioca flour, stirring quickly to mix the batter. It should thicken from the residual heat of the saucepan. Add the remaining tapioca flour. Stir until it becomes a batter. Generously dust a work surface with tapioca flour and pour the batter onto it. Allow it to cool for 1 or 2 minutes and begin to knead the dough together into a ball. Use a dough scraper because the batter will be extremely sticky. Dust more tapioca flour as you cut the dough into 8 portions and cover with plastic wrap.

3. Take one portion and roll it into a log approximately ⅜-inch thick. Using the dough scraper, cut small pieces and roll them into balls. Transfer the tapioca balls to a baking sheet generously dusted with tapioca flour. Repeat with the rest of the portions. Once all the tapioca balls have been formed, shake off excess tapioca flour and store in freezer-safe bags in the freezer for at least an hour.

bubble tea
continued

4. To cook the tapioca balls, bring a large pot of water to a full boil. Using a spatula, stir the water to create some movement before adding in uncooked, frozen tapioca balls. Cook for 20 minutes, stirring occasionally to prevent sticking. Remove the pot from the heat and allow the tapioca balls to sit in the water for an additional 15 minutes to heat through. Drain and rinse the tapioca balls with cold water.

5. Using a fine-mesh strainer, scoop the tapioca balls into a large bowl. Create a quick syrup by mixing ⅓ cup dark brown sugar, the kief-infused honey, and ¼ cup hot water in a small bowl. Pour it into the bowl of tapioca balls and stir to coat.

6. Now the infused tapioca balls are ready to use with your favorite hot or cold milk tea.

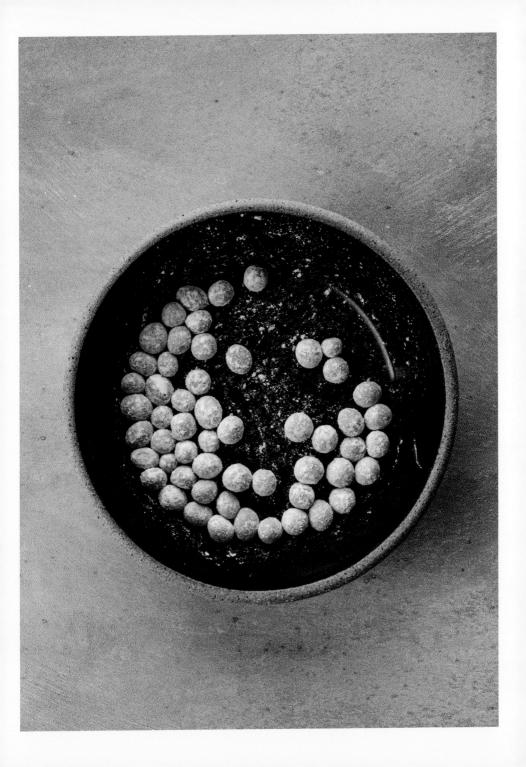

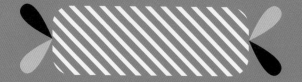

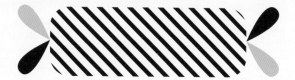

2

soft caramels & nougats

For those who are new to candy making, soft caramels and nougats are a great way to practice the basics of using a candy thermometer and understanding your kitchen setup's idiosyncrasies. You may discover that you need a heavier saucepan or that your stove runs hotter than other stoves.

This chapter is a bit more forgiving than the "Hard & Brittle" chapter (page 93) and offers you a chance to iron out the kinks in your workflow.

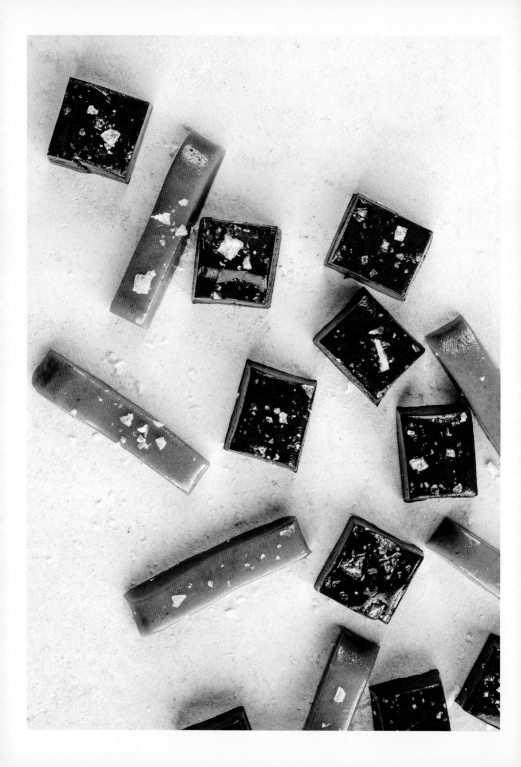

salted mocha caramels

Makes 64 pieces

Active Time
1½ hours

Inactive Time
4 hours

Ingredients
½ cup unsalted butter
4 tablespoons
Cannabis-Infused Butter
(page 38)
1 cup light corn syrup
2 cups granulated sugar
4 ounces unsweetened
chocolate, chopped
1 cup heavy whipping
cream
1 teaspoon vanilla
extract
1 tablespoon instant
coffee granules
2 teaspoons hot water
Maldon salt, to finish

Special Equipment
8-inch square baking
pan
medium heavy-
bottomed saucepan
candy or instant-read
thermometer

I love a good sweet and salty treat, and this is one of my favorite recipes in this book. These Salted Mocha Caramels are dark, creamy, and so irresistible. The type of instant coffee you use is important when making these caramels, so be sure to select one that you also enjoy drinking.

1. Line an 8-inch square baking pan with a sheet of parchment paper. Crease the corners along the inside edges and leave a 1-inch overhang on each side of the pan. Lightly coat with nonstick spray.

2. In a medium heavy-bottomed saucepan over medium heat, add the butter, cannabis-infused butter, light corn syrup, granulated sugar, unsweetened chocolate, and heavy whipping cream. Stir until the butter and sugar have melted, about 5 minutes.

3. Decrease the heat to medium low and clip a candy thermometer to the saucepan, stirring occasionally to prevent the bottom from burning. While the caramel is cooking, add the vanilla extract, instant coffee granules, and hot water to a small bowl and stir to combine.

4. Once the temperature of the caramel registers 242°F (117°C) on the candy thermometer, about 30 minutes, remove from the heat and gently stir in the coffee mixture. Beware of steam as you stir.

5. Pour into the prepared pan. Cool for 30 minutes, then sprinkle flaky Maldon salt over the surface of the caramel. Allow to cool completely, about 4 hours.

6. Remove the caramels from the pan by pulling on the parchment paper. Wipe a sharp kitchen knife with nonstick cooking spray. Cut the caramels into 1-inch squares and wrap them with candy wrappers. Store in an airtight container or in the fridge for up to 2 months.

miso butterscotch caramels

Makes 32 to 64 pieces

Active Time
1½ hours

Inactive Time
4 hours

Ingredients

½ cup unsalted butter

4 tablespoons Cannabis-Infused Butter (page 38)

1 cup light corn syrup

2¼ cups firmly packed light brown sugar

1 cup heavy whipping cream

¼ cup water

1 teaspoon vanilla extract

2 tablespoons shiro miso

2 teaspoons hot water

Maldon salt, to finish

Special Equipment

8-inch square baking pan

medium heavy-bottomed saucepan

candy or instant-read thermometer

This is another winning sweet and salty combination: the flavor of butterscotch mixes with the umami from miso to create these rich and luscious caramels. There are different types of miso paste at the grocery store; be sure to pick up shiro miso (or white miso), which has a milder, sweeter flavor and lends itself nicely to candies and baked goods. These caramels are wonderful on their own but would also be delicious chopped up and baked into a kitchen sink cookie.

1. Line an 8-inch square baking pan with parchment paper. Crease the corners along the inside edges and leave a 1-inch overhang on each side of the pan. Lightly coat with nonstick spray.

2. In a medium heavy-bottomed saucepan over medium heat, add the butter, cannabis-infused butter, light corn syrup, light brown sugar, heavy whipping cream, and water. Stir until the butter and sugar have melted, about 5 minutes.

3. Decrease the heat to medium low and clip a candy thermometer to the saucepan, stirring occasionally to prevent the bottom from burning.

4. While the butterscotch is cooking, add the vanilla extract, shiro miso, and hot water to a small bowl and stir to combine.

5. Once the temperature of the butterscotch registers 242°F (117°C) on the candy thermometer, about 30 minutes, remove from the heat and gently stir in the miso mixture. Beware of steam as you stir.

6. Pour the mixture into the prepared baking pan. Cool for 30 minutes, then sprinkle flaky Maldon salt over the surface of the caramel and gently press in

with gloved hands. Allow to cool completely, about 4 hours.

7. Remove caramels from the pan by pulling on the parchment paper. Wipe a sharp kitchen knife with nonstick cooking spray.

8. Cut into 2 x 1-inch rectangles or 1-inch squares and wrap with candy wrappers. Store in an airtight container or in the fridge for up to 2 months.

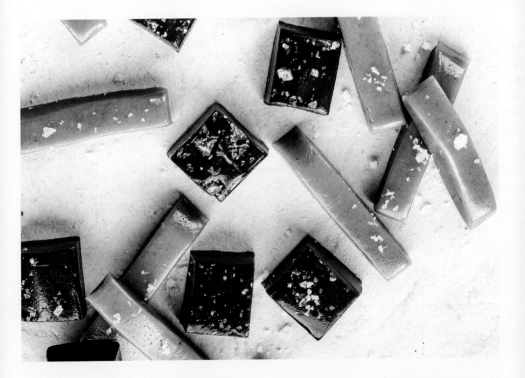

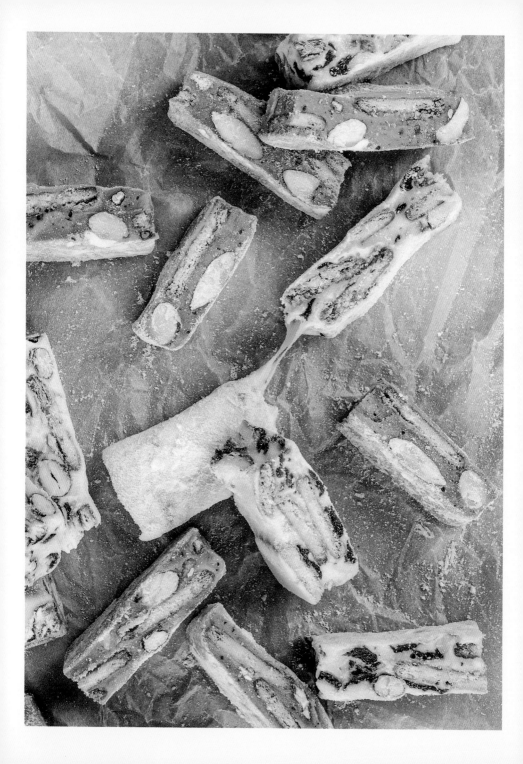

snowflake crisp nougat

Makes 32 pieces

Active Time
10 minutes

Inactive Time
1 hour

Ingredients
4 tablespoons unsalted butter
4 tablespoons Cannabis-Infused Butter (page 38)
1 (10-ounce) bag marshmallows
1 cup milk powder

Flavoring Suggestions
4 teaspoons culinary-grade matcha powder
¾ cup whole almonds, toasted
1 cup dried cranberries
130 g tea biscuits (approximately 1½ cups)

Final Dusting
1 tablespoon milk powder
3 tablespoons powdered sugar

Special Equipment
8-inch square baking pan
large heavy-bottomed saucepan

This particular treat is near and dear to my heart. My late grandparents used to send care packages filled with milk nougats to us from Taiwan, where these candies originated. Traditionally these nougats are made with roasted peanuts or dried fruit, but these days there are a variety of flavors, such as matcha, strawberry, salted egg yolk, and even scallion. Some also contain crackers or tea biscuits for an extra-crispy and flaky textural component. My parents were excited to work on this recipe with me, and we're sharing two flavors because we couldn't decide which was tastier.

1. Line an 8-inch square baking pan with parchment paper.

2. In a large heavy-bottomed saucepan over medium-low heat, melt the butter and cannabis-infused butter. Add the marshmallows and stir frequently with a silicone spatula until completely melted. Then stir in the dry milk powder and mix until combined.

3. Remove from the heat and add in your choice of flavorings, gently folding the ingredients in with a spatula until the mixture is coated in marshmallow.

Matcha Almond Snowflake Crisp Nougat Option: Add the matcha powder first and mix until the sticky batter is uniform in color. Then add the toasted almonds and whole tea biscuits. The tea biscuits will crumble as you compress the nougat.

Cranberry Almond Snowflake Crisp Nougat Option: Add the toasted almonds, dried cranberries, and whole tea biscuits. The tea biscuits will crumble as you compress the nougat.

4. Transfer the mixture into the prepared baking pan and cover the top with a piece of parchment paper.

snowflake crisp nougat

continued

Using the palm of your hand, firmly press down to compress the nougat into an even, solid slab.

5. Cool completely, about an hour, before unmolding. In a small bowl, mix the dry milk powder and powdered sugar. Pour into a fine-mesh sieve and lightly dust each side of the slab with the dusting powder. Slice into 1 x 2-inch rectangles. Wrap in candy wrappers.

6. Store in an airtight container for up to 2 weeks.

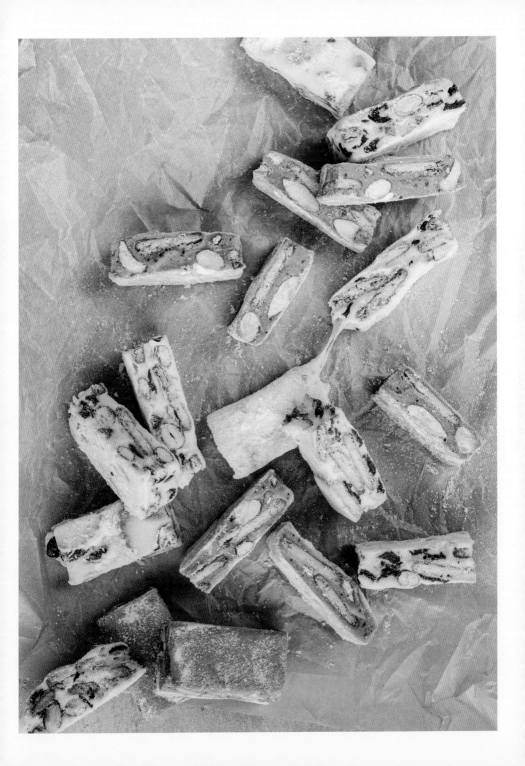

creamy milk candy

Makes 24 pieces

Active Time
25 minutes

Inactive Time
1 hour

Ingredients

¾ cup whole milk

2 tablespoons Cannabis-Infused Butter (page 38), softened

2 tablespoons unsalted butter, softened

¼ cup light corn syrup

½ cup granulated sugar

2 tablespoons tapioca flour

1½ cups plus 1 tablespoon milk powder, divided

½ teaspoon vanilla extract

3 tablespoons powdered sugar

Special Equipment

medium heavy-bottomed saucepan

fine-mesh sieve

instant-read thermometer

There are a million varieties of creamy milk candies in different cultures around the world. Some are fudgy, some are soft and creamy, and some are chewy and taffy-like. Regardless of texture, candy making is a great way to use up milk before it spoils. This cannabis-infused version is creamy with a soft chew.

1. Line a baking sheet with parchment paper. Lightly coat with nonstick spray.

2. Combine the milk, both butters, light corn syrup, and sugar in a medium heavy-bottomed saucepan. Using a fine-mesh sieve, sift in the tapioca flour and 1½ cups of the dry milk powder to prevent clumps. Whisk until the mixture is completely uniform.

3. Turn the heat to medium and stir with a silicone spatula for 5 minutes. Reduce the heat to medium low, stirring constantly to prevent burning. Remove from the heat when the instant-read thermometer registers between 235°F and 240°F (113°C and 116°C), 10 to 15 minutes.

4. Stir in the vanilla extract. Pour onto the prepared baking sheet and shape into a 6 x 6-inch square with the silicone spatula. Cool completely, about an hour.

5. In a small bowl, mix together the remaining 1 tablespoon of dry milk powder and the powdered sugar; then, using a fine-mesh sieve, dust both sides of the milk candy slab with this mixture. Slice the slab into 1 x 1½-inch rectangles. Wrap in wax candy wrappers. Store in an airtight container.

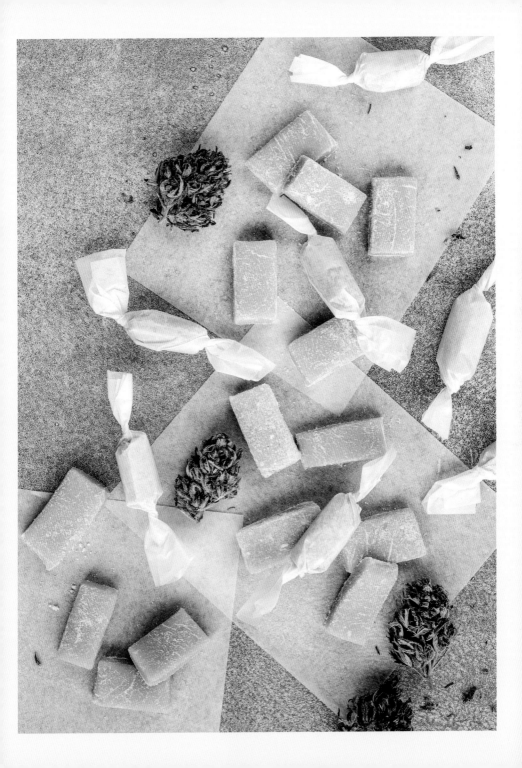

chocolate turtles

Makes 12 pieces

Active Time
45 minutes

Ingredients

60 pecan halves (approximately 5 ounces), roasted

25 baking caramel squares

1 tablespoon Cannabis-Infused Butter (page 38)

2 tablespoons heavy cream

1¼ cups dark or milk chocolate baking chips

1 tablespoon cannabis-infused coconut oil (page 40)

Maldon salt, to finish

Special Equipment
double boiler

The smell of roasted pecans instantly brings me back to my childhood in Texas. The combination of chocolate, caramel, and pecans feels so Southern to me and is probably why I adore chocolate turtles so much. Quality chocolate makes the difference here. I like a bitter, dark chocolate from Guittard for the final coating to cut through the sweetness of the caramel. A sprinkle of flaky Maldon salt adds a delicate crunch and elegance to this treat.

1. Arrange 15 stacked mounds of roasted pecans, 4 pecans per stack, on a parchment-lined baking sheet.

2. Add 3 inches of water to the bottom pan of your double boiler and set the heat to medium. Once the water comes to a boil, set the top double boiler pan or bowl on the bottom pan and add the baking caramel squares, cannabis-infused butter, and heavy cream. Stir every minute or so with a silicone spatula until the caramel is completely melted and silky smooth, 10 to 15 minutes.

3. Spoon 2 teaspoons of the warm caramel onto each pecan stack and set aside to harden.

4. Add 2 inches of water to the bottom pan of your double boiler and set the heat to medium. Once the water comes to a boil, set the top double boiler pan or bowl on the bottom pan and add the chocolate baking chips and cannabis-infused coconut oil. Stir every minute or so with a silicone spatula until the chocolate is completely melted and uniform.

5. Spoon the chocolate over the top of each pecan stack to cover the caramel. Finish with a light sprinkle of flaky Maldon salt on top of each turtle. Store in an airtight container in the fridge or freezer.

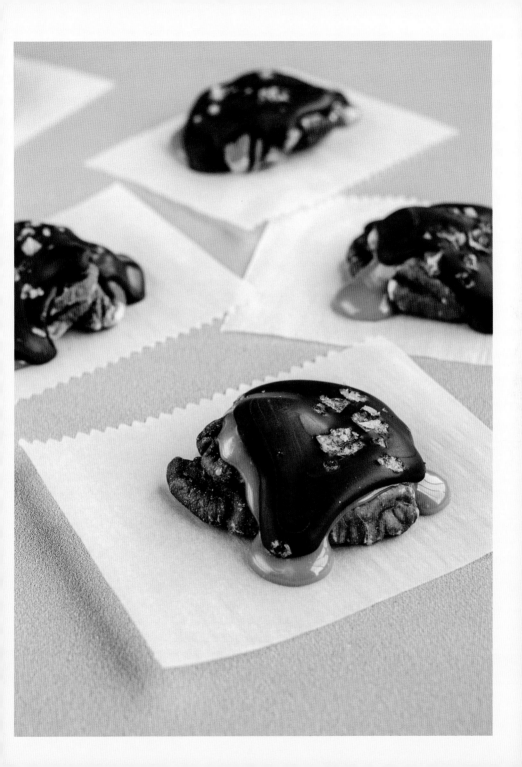

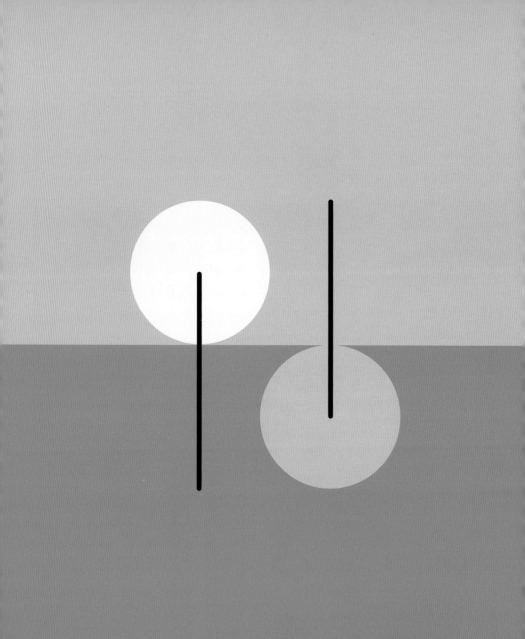

3

hard & brittle

Sound the alarms! This chapter has been unofficially dubbed "The Danger Zone." Before proceeding, please brush up on the Candy-Making Tips and Safety Notes (page 22) to make sure you are good to go.

My final recommendation is to do an uninfused trial run of the recipe before you use your precious cannabis infusion. Sugar work is fussy, and different variables in your kitchen can affect the end results—so practice first!

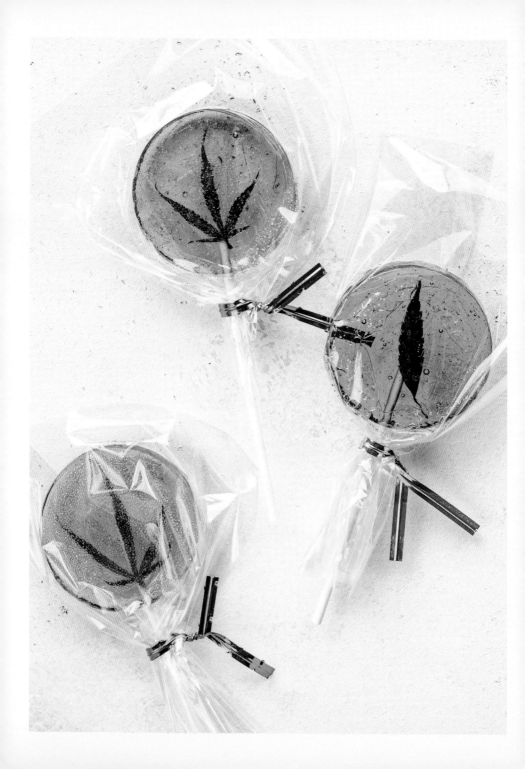

sugar leaf lollipops

Makes 8 lollipops

Active Time
40 minutes

Inactive Time
15 minutes

Ingredients

¾ cup granulated sugar

½ cup light corn syrup

¼ cup water

1 to 2 drops food coloring

¼ to ½ teaspoon super-strength candy flavoring of your choice

3 teaspoons Cannabis-Infused Tincture (page 43)

cannabis or hemp sugar leaves (optional)

edible flowers

Special Equipment

medium heavy-bottomed saucepan

silicone spatula

candy or instant-read thermometer

2-inch lollipop molds

lollipop sticks

tweezers

heat-resistant kitchen gloves

If you grow cannabis or hemp at home, lollipops are a fun way to preserve the beautiful small sugar leaves from your trimmings. As mentioned in the chapter opener, hard candies can be challenging, and different variables can affect your results. I've made these lollipops many times, and every once in a while I will ruin a batch. I would recommend a trial run or two without using your cannabis-infused tincture and sugar leaves so you can get acquainted with your workflow.

1. Lightly grease eight 2-inch lollipop molds with nonstick cooking spray and wipe with a paper towel. Insert lollipop sticks. Set aside.

2. Add the granulated sugar, light corn syrup, and water to a medium heavy-bottomed saucepan and mix well. Place over medium-low heat and clip a candy thermometer to the saucepan. Stir with a silicone spatula until the sugar has completely dissolved.

3. Once the mixture comes to a simmer, decrease the temperature to low so the sugar doesn't brown. Do not stir until the temperature registers 300°F (149°C) on the candy thermometer, about 30 minutes. Immediately remove from the heat and allow to rest for a few seconds while the bubbling slows down. Stir in the food coloring, super-strength candy flavoring, and cannabis-infused tincture. Beware of steam as you stir.

4. Wearing heat-resistant kitchen gloves, gently spoon the mixture into a prepared lollipop mold until half full. Then use tweezers to arrange the cannabis or sugar leaves, if using, and edible flowers. Continue to fill the molds with the mixture until full. Allow to cool completely, about 15 minutes. Unmold and wrap in plastic.

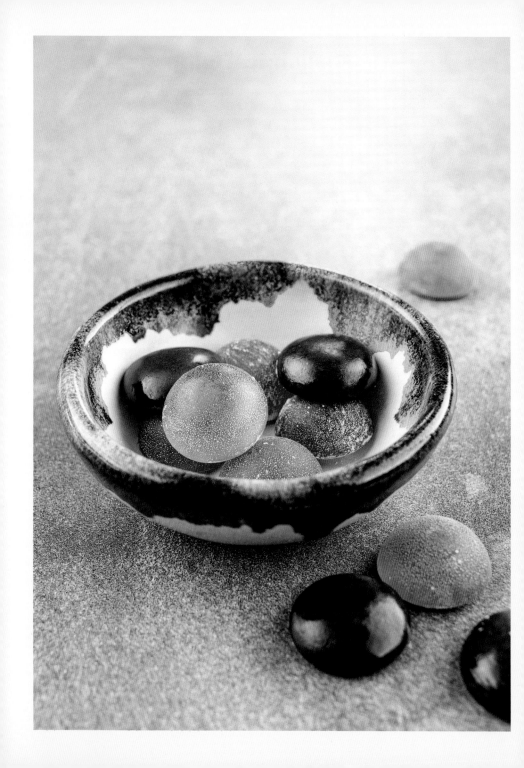

honey elderberry lozenges

Makes 10 (1.18-inch) round lozenges

Active Time
25 minutes

Inactive Time
1 hour

Ingredients

¼ cup plus 2 tablespoons honey

2 tablespoons Kief-Infused Honey (page 42)

2 tablespoons elderberry syrup

Final Dusting

2 tablespoons cornstarch

1 tablespoon powdered sugar

Special Equipment

small heavy-bottomed saucepan

candy or instant-read thermometer

silicone lozenge mold

heat-resistant kitchen gloves

Made with simple ingredients, this lozenge is a good one to keep around during cold and flu season. In several small studies, researchers have found that elderberry could potentially help alleviate cold symptoms in a shorter amount of time. The addition of honey, a natural humectant (meaning it can retain moisture), makes this an effective cough drop. For this same reason, you'll want a final dusting of cornstarch to keep the lozenges from sticking together.

1. Lightly grease the silicone lozenge mold with nonstick cooking spray and wipe with a paper towel.

2. Fill a large mixing bowl with ice and water. Set aside.

3. Add the honey and kief-infused honey to a small heavy-bottomed saucepan. Place over medium heat and clip a candy thermometer to the saucepan.

4. Do not stir until the temperature registers 275°F (135°C) on the candy thermometer. Add the elderberry syrup and let the temperature rise to 300°F (149°C). Honey burns quickly so immediately remove from the heat and submerge the bottom of the saucepan in the ice bath to stop the cooking. Do not allow any water to enter the saucepan. Stir until the bubbles subside.

5. Wearing heat-resistant kitchen gloves, gently spoon the mixture into the prepared lozenge mold and allow to cool completely, about an hour. Unmold and toss in a light dusting of cornstarch and powdered sugar before storing in an airtight container in the fridge.

sour yuzu drops

Active Time
25 minutes

Inactive Time
1 hour

___

Ingredients

2 tablespoons water

¼ cup plus 2 table-spoons granulated sugar

2 tablespoons light corn syrup

¾ teaspoon citric acid, divided

¼ teaspoon yuzu extract oil or lemon extract oil

2 teaspoons Cannabis-Infused Tincture (page 43)

2 drops yellow food coloring (optional)

¼ cup powdered sugar

Special Equipment

small heavy-bottomed saucepan

silicone spatula

pastry brush

candy or instant-read thermometer

Yuzu seems to be experiencing a consistent rise in popularity. It's a darling little citrus commonly used in Japanese cuisine, and the aroma is exquisite. The zest is sweet, floral, and reminiscent of grapefruit and mandarin orange. Yuzu is quite the prized ingredient, which makes it rather pricey. Lemon extract oil will do the trick as well if that's easier to find.

1. Fill a large mixing bowl with ice and water. Set aside.

2. Add the water, granulated sugar, and light corn syrup to a small heavy-bottomed saucepan and mix well. Place over medium heat and clip a candy thermometer to the saucepan. Stir with a silicone spatula until the sugar has completely dissolved. Dip a pastry brush into hot water and brush down the sides of the saucepan to prevent crystallization.

3. Once the mixture comes to a simmer, decrease the temperature to medium low. Do not stir until the temperature registers 300°F (149°C) on the candy thermometer, about 10 minutes. Immediately remove from the heat and submerge the bottom of the saucepan in the ice bath to stop the cooking. Do not allow any water to enter the saucepan.

4. Gently stir in ½ teaspoon of the citric acid, the yuzu extract oil or lemon extract oil, the cannabis-infused tincture, and the food coloring, if using, until uniform in color. Spoon into a prepared candy mold and allow to cool completely, about an hour.

5. Prepare the sour powder by mixing the remaining ¼ teaspoon of citric acid and the powdered sugar in a small mixing bowl. Unmold the cooled candies and toss them in the sour powder to lightly coat. Store in an airtight container.

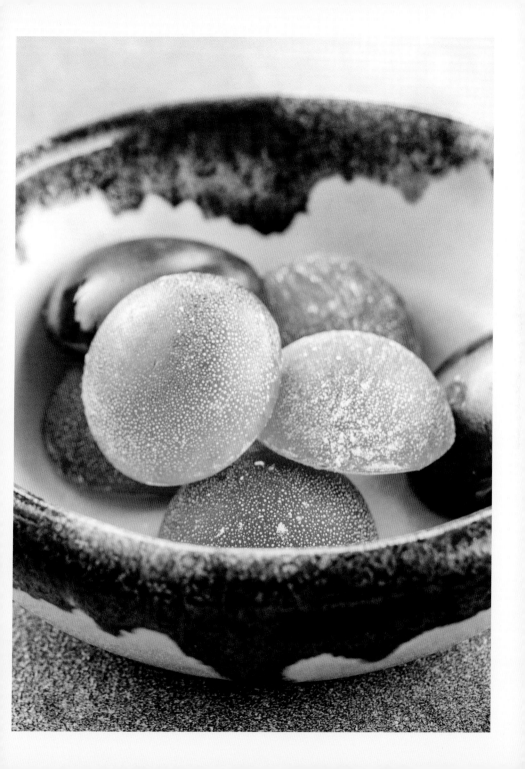

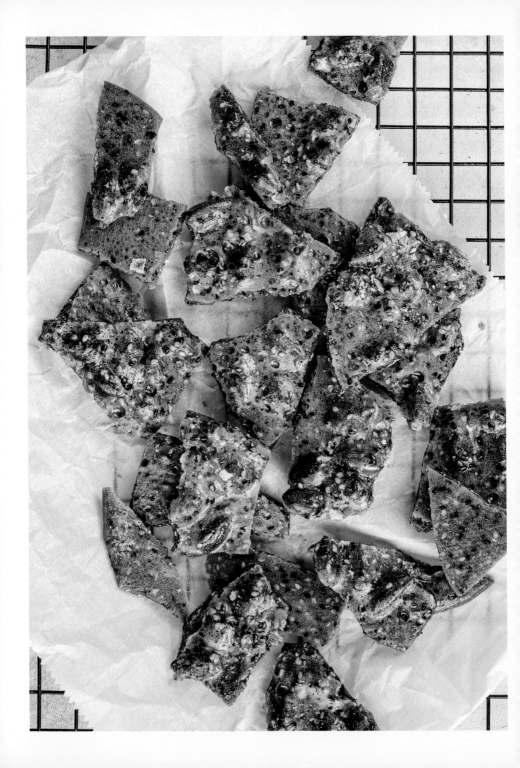

honeycomb brittle with almonds & sesame seeds

Makes 24 pieces

Active Time
25 minutes

Inactive Time
2 hours

Ingredients

1¼ cups granulated sugar

¼ cup Kief-Infused Honey (page 42)

¼ cup light corn syrup

¼ cup water

1¼ cups whole almonds, toasted

¼ cup black sesame seeds

¼ cup white sesame seeds

1 tablespoon unsalted butter, melted

½ teaspoon vanilla extract

1 teaspoon baking soda

Maldon salt, to finish

Special Equipment

medium heavy-bottomed saucepan

silicone spatula

candy or instant-read thermometer

silicone baking mat

heat-resistant kitchen gloves

This is a recipe that has yet to make it onto my blog because it's my number one go-to giftable treat every holiday season. I didn't want to give away all my secrets, but I couldn't resist sharing with you. Roasted almonds, mixed sesame seeds, and flaky sea salt are a wonderful combination and add a rich nuttiness that balances the sweetness of the brittle.

1. Prepare a baking sheet with a silicone mat and set aside.

2. In a medium heavy-bottomed saucepan over medium-high heat, add the sugar, kief-infused honey, light corn syrup, and water. Clip a candy thermometer to the saucepan.

3. Stir constantly until the mixture comes to a boil. Then reduce the heat to medium. When the temperature registers 275°F (135°C), mix in the almonds and sesame seeds, stirring to coat.

4. When the temperature reaches 300°F (149°C) on the candy thermometer, immediately remove the mixture from the heat. Add the butter, vanilla extract, and baking soda and quickly stir the mixture as it expands in size. Beware of steam as you stir.

5. Wearing heat-resistant kitchen gloves, pour the brittle mixture onto the prepared baking sheet and spread it thin using a silicone spatula. Sprinkle Maldon salt across the surface and let it cool completely, about 2 hours.

6. Break the brittle into pieces and package it in candy bags or store in airtight containers.

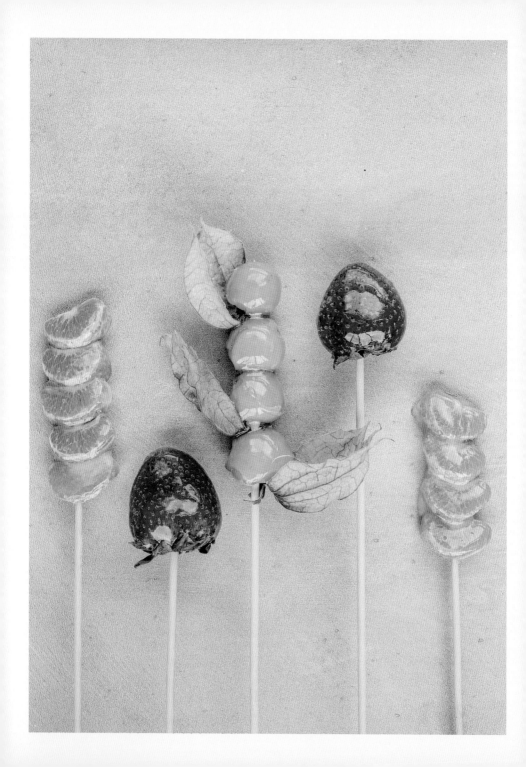

candied fruit

Active Time
25 minutes

Ingredients
1 pound fresh fruit

1¾ cups granulated sugar

¼ cup Cannabis-Infused Sugar (page 44)

1 cup water

Special Equipment
silicone baking mat

10-inch bamboo skewers

silicone spatula

small heavy-bottomed saucepan

candy or instant-read thermometer

You'll often find these shiny, candy-coated fruit, called tanghulu, while strolling through the night markets in Taiwan or China. Street vendors will dip fresh fruit, like strawberries, grapes, and tangerines, in molten sugar to create a thin candy shell that shatters as you bite into it. Be sure the surface of your fruit is dry for the candy coating to stick. This recipe requires precise temperature control and that you work swiftly to coat the fruit. Practice a few times with non-infused sugar until you get used to the motions.

1. Prepare a baking sheet with a silicone baking mat and set aside.

2. Wash your fruit of choice and pat dry with a paper towel. Add 1 to 3 pieces of the fruit to a bamboo skewer and set aside.

3. In a small heavy-bottomed saucepan over medium-high heat, combine the granulated sugar, cannabis-infused sugar, and water. Clip a candy thermometer to the saucepan.

4. Stir until the mixture comes to a boil. Then reduce the heat to medium. When the temperature reaches 300°F (149°C) on the candy thermometer, about 5 minutes, immediately remove from the heat.

5. Working quickly and carefully, dip the skewered fruit into the mixture and turn to fully coat. Set on the prepared baking sheet to cool and harden. The candy coating won't last long as the fruit releases moisture so enjoy within an hour.

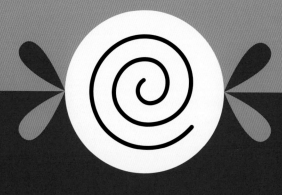

4

sugar alternatives

I won't say they're healthier, but if you're hungry for treats using sweeteners that are less processed, here are some ideas that don't skimp on flavor.

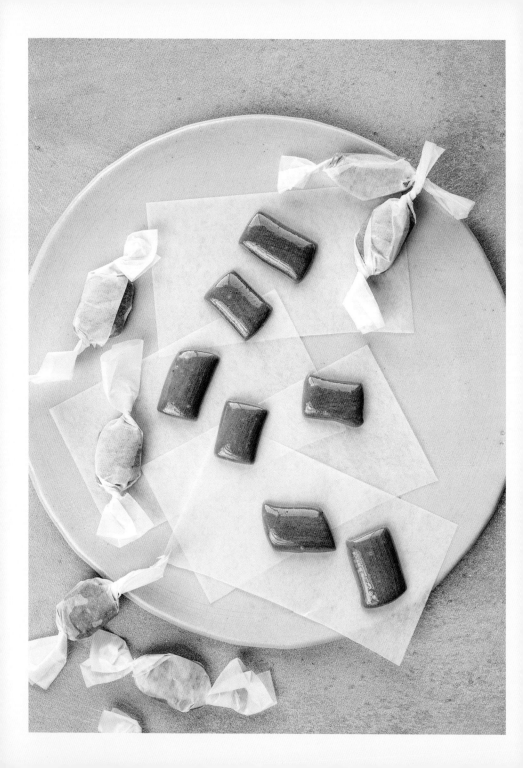

ginger honey chews

Active Time
45 minutes

Ingredients

¼ cup ginger juice, fresh

¾ cup honey

1 tablespoon Cannabis-Infused Tincture (page 43)

nonstick cooking spray or neutral cooking oil

Special Equipment

silicone baking mat

small heavy-bottomed saucepan

candy or instant-read thermometer

silicone spatula

dough scraper

Late at night, you will probably catch me bingeing old-fashioned, candy-pulling ASMR videos on YouTube. It's incredibly satisfying to watch, and it's equally enjoyable to make at home. This recipe uses fresh ginger juice, which you can blitz in a blender or food processor and pass through a fine-mesh strainer. Since candy pulling requires precise temperature control and manual labor, I recommend practicing once or twice without the cannabis tincture to figure out the kinks. And don't be afraid to be liberal when greasing your hands during the pulling and aerating process!

1. Prepare a baking sheet with a silicone baking mat or parchment paper. Lightly coat with nonstick cooking spray.

2. In a small heavy-bottomed saucepan over medium heat, bring the ginger juice and honey to a boil, stirring until the honey dissolves. Clip a candy thermometer to the saucepan.

3. Reduce the heat to medium low and stop stirring. When the temperature reaches 275°F (135°C) on the candy thermometer, about 15 minutes, immediately remove from the heat and stir in the cannabis-infused tincture with a silicone spatula. Beware of steam as you stir.

4. Pour the mixture onto the prepared baking sheet. Let it rest for 5 minutes until it is cool enough to handle. Spray your hands and the dough scraper with nonstick cooking spray and begin to work the ginger chew into a ball. Stretch the ball into a long rope and fold it over on itself. Continue to stretch and fold until the color of the ginger chew turns from amber to an opaque, golden tan and the consistency is taffy-like, about 10 minutes. Using the dough scraper coated in nonstick cooking spray, cut the chew into 1 x ½-inch rectangles. Wrap in wax candy wrappers. Store in an airtight container or in the fridge.

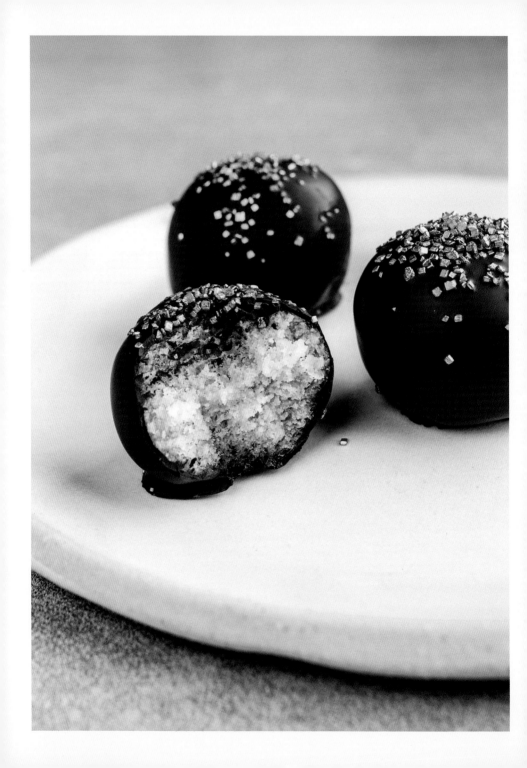

marzipan truffles

Makes 24 truffles

Active Time
1½ hours

Inactive Time
1 hour

Ingredients
1½ cups almond flour
½ cup monk fruit sweetener
¼ cup Kief-Infused Honey (page 42)
1½ teaspoons almond extract
½ tablespoon water, if needed
8.5 ounces unsweetened chocolate chips
1 tablespoon cannabis-infused coconut oil (page 40)
Edible glitter or sprinkles, to finish

Special Equipment
double boiler
stand mixer

The dessert possibilities are endless with this cannabis-infused marzipan recipe. Chocolate coating, for one, is an easy way to make your marzipan into bite-size truffles. Now imagine sculpting marzipan fruit to decorate your pastries, marzipan yule logs, or even an infused Christmas stollen!

1. Add the almond flour and monk fruit sweetener to the bowl of the stand mixer fitted with the paddle attachment. Mix on low to break up any clumps. Add the kief-infused honey and almond extract and mix on low to combine into a dough. If the marzipan is still dry, add a teaspoon of water and continue to blend.

2. Turn the marzipan onto a work surface and knead until the dough is stiff. Form it into a 10-inch-long log, wrap in plastic wrap, and refrigerate for an hour.

3. Cut the chilled marzipan into 24 equal pieces and roll into balls. Set on a wire rack with a baking sheet underneath.

4. To make the chocolate coating, add 2 inches of water to the bottom pan of a double boiler and set the heat to medium. Once the water comes to a boil, set the top double boiler pan or bowl on the bottom pan and add the chocolate chips and cannabis-infused coconut oil. Stir every minute or so with a silicone spatula until the chocolate is completely melted and uniform in texture.

5. Gently spoon the melted chocolate over the truffles until they are covered. Top with glitter or sprinkles. Store in the fridge.

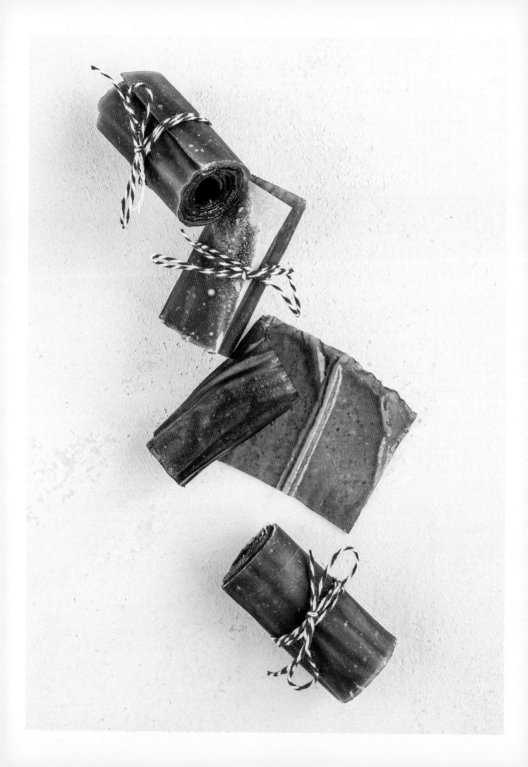

tropical fruit leather rolls

Makes 6 fruit rolls

Active Time
15 minutes

Inactive Time
5 hours

Ingredients

3 Ataulfo mangoes

½ Hawaiian papaya

1 tablespoon Kief-Infused Honey (page 42)

1 teaspoon Rapid Set HM pectin

juice of 1 lime

This recipe is inspired by my friend Andres, who I lovingly call Papaya Papi. His obsession with tropical fruits rubbed off on me, and I found my fridge full of papayas and mangoes this summer. Many made their way into my morning yogurt bowls, but they were also pureed for fruit leather snacks. If mangoes and papayas are not in season, use whatever fruit or berries you'd like as long as the pureed fruit yields 2 cups. A touch of pectin will give the fruit leather a glossy sheen and keep it pliable.

1. Line a baking sheet with parchment paper and set aside.

2. Preheat the oven or dehydrator to 165°F (75°C).

3. Prep the mangoes and papaya by removing the skin, pit, and seeds. Add the flesh to a food processor with the kief-infused honey and pectin. Puree until uniform.

4. Transfer the fruit mixture to a saucepan and bring to a simmer over medium heat, about 5 minutes. Remove from the heat and add the lime juice. Mix well.

5. Pour the mixture onto the prepared baking sheet and spread thinly and evenly using a spatula.

6. Place the sheet with the fruit leather mixture in the oven or dehydrator to dehydrate for 4 to 5 hours. When finished, the fruit leather should be dry to the touch with a glossy sheen.

7. Remove from the oven or dehydrator and trim the edges of the parchment paper on all sides. Roll up the fruit leather, parchment paper included, and cut into 6 pieces. Store in an airtight container in the fridge.

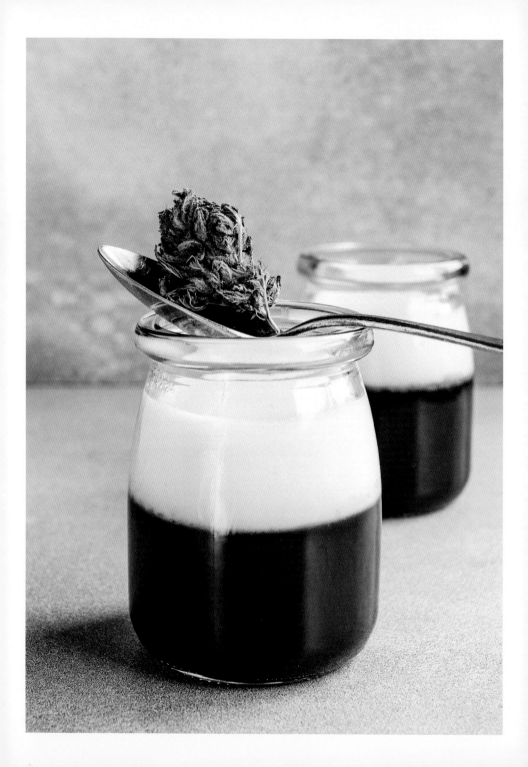

blueberries & cream jellies

Active Time
20 minutes

Inactive Time
20 to 30 minutes

Ingredients

1 cup frozen wild blueberries

3½ tablespoons monk fruit sweetener, divided

¾ cup water

1¾ teaspoons agar-agar powder, divided

1 tablespoon Cannabis-Infused Tincture (page 43)

½ cup coconut milk

Special Equipment

fine-mesh strainer

silicone mold

mason jars (optional)

Wild blueberries may be smaller than the conventional blueberry, but they pack significantly more flavor and sweetness, which is why I always have a bag in my freezer for morning smoothies or jellies. These duotone jellies look lovely in mason jars or as little cubes for a quick afternoon snack. Made with agar-agar and coconut milk, this treat is completely vegan friendly.

1. In a food processor, blend the frozen blueberries, ½ tablespoon monk fruit sweetener, and water together. Using a fine-mesh strainer, strain the juice into a small saucepan and add 1¼ teaspoons of the agar-agar powder. Whisk to combine.

2. Turn the heat to medium and bring the mixture to a boil for 5 minutes to activate the agar-agar. Remove from the heat and add in the cannabis-infused tincture. Stir until uniform. Pour into a measuring cup with a spout and gently fill the silicone molds or mason jars halfway. Set in the fridge for 5 minutes to solidify.

3. Add the coconut milk, remaining 3 tablespoons of monk fruit sweetener, and ½ teaspoon agar-agar powder to a small saucepan and whisk to combine. Turn the heat to medium and bring the mixture to a simmer to activate the agar-agar, about 3 minutes. Remove from the heat and pour through a fine-mesh strainer into a measuring cup with a spout. This will remove the bubbles from the cream.

4. Check to see that the blueberry layer has solidified on the surface—it should be soft and jiggly to the touch so that the cream layer will bind to it. Gently fill the silicone molds or mason jars the rest of the way.

5. Chill the jellies in the fridge until firm, 20 to 30 minutes. Store in the fridge.

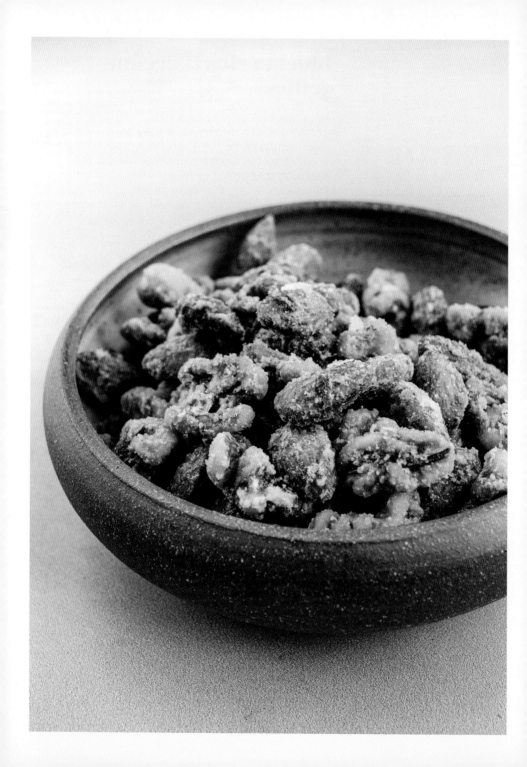

lemon rosemary party nuts

Makes 8 servings

Active Time
30 minutes

Ingredients

4 cups raw assorted nuts

2 tablespoons Cannabis-Infused Butter (page 38), melted

juice of 1 large lemon

1 large egg white

½ cup monk fruit sweetener

½ teaspoon vanilla extract

2 tablespoons chopped rosemary, fresh

1 teaspoon kosher salt

zest of 1 large lemon

Maldon salt, to finish

Liven up your next dinner event with these crunchy party nuts that taste like lemon rosemary shortbread. Lemon and rosemary are aromatics often seen during the holidays, so this recipe is a great way to use up leftover ingredients. It also stores well for gift giving. I enjoy this bright, herbaceous flavor combination with almonds and walnuts, but feel free to use whatever nuts you have on hand and go nuts!

1. Line a baking sheet with parchment paper and set aside.

2. Preheat the oven to 300°F (149°C).

3. In a large mixing bowl, coat the assorted raw nuts in the melted cannabis-infused butter and lemon juice. Set aside to marinate for 10 minutes.

4. In a separate mixing bowl, beat the egg white until stiff peaks form. Add the monk fruit sweetener and continue to beat for another 10 seconds, until the sweetener is thoroughly mixed in.

5. In the bowl of nuts, add the vanilla extract, chopped rosemary, and kosher salt and mix well. Gently fold in the fluffy egg-white mixture until the nuts are coated.

6. Spread the coated nuts evenly on the prepared baking sheet. Bake for 10 minutes, then remove from the oven and add the lemon zest. Stir with a spatula to evenly coat the nuts. Return them to the oven and bake for an additional 5 minutes. Remove the nuts from the oven and sprinkle with flaky Maldon salt.

7. Cool the nuts completely before storing them in an airtight container.

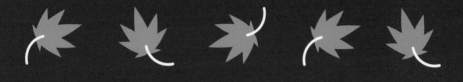

educational resources

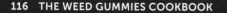

ardent

At Ardent, we focus on the vision of "what can be" and strive to develop innovative technology and products to bring the power of cannabis to the individual. Ardent fully celebrates the plant, giving patients and consumers access as well as the freedom to accurately dose and control what products—edibles, tinctures, and beyond—are going into their bodies. By providing both the precision tools and educational resources, we've helped eliminate intimidation and guesswork from the DIY process.

—Shanel Lindsay, Founder & CEO

Visit *ArdentCannabis.com*

do the pot

How to Do the Pot is an audio-first education platform demystifying cannabis for women. We are on a mission to inspire women to feel confident in their choices about cannabis for health, well-being, and fun. Check out the podcast wherever you listen!

—Ellen Lee Scanlon, CEO & Cofounder

Visit *DoThePot.com*

grow it from home

You can join a community of gardeners across the US successfully growing cannabis at home. Grow It From Home provides plants, seeds, and garden accessories, shipping direct from our USDA Organic certified farm to your doorstep. It's just as easy to grow as a tomato, and it grows like a weed!

—Emily Gogol, PhD, Head Gardener

Visit *GrowItFromHome.com*

inclusivebase

"

Inclusivebase was created in the hopes that people would utilize it to shop responsibly and support Black, Indigenous, and People of Color (BIPOC) communities when it comes to cannabis. When we look at the history of cannabis and where consumption and farming practices originated, it's hard to ignore that BIPOC cultures contributed greatly to the knowledge and progress around this plant. There are hundreds of plant-touching and ancillary businesses in the Inclusivebase directory, as well as education and advocacy-base organizations. Please encourage your friends to shop and support BIPOC!

—Kieryn Wang, Inclusivebase Co-Collaborator

Visit *Inclusivebase.com*

last prisoner project

"

The Last Prisoner Project is a national, nonpartisan not-for-profit that works to end America's discriminatory and counterproductive policy of cannabis criminalization, as well as to repair the harms of this unjust and ineffective crusade. Through intervention, awareness, and advocacy, we seek to secure "full freedom" for the millions of people who have needlessly suffered as a result of marijuana prohibition.

—Sarah Gersten, Executive Director and General Counsel, Last Prisoner Project

Visit *LastPrisonerProject.org*

the herb somm

"

The Herb Somm is a culinary-meets-cannabis blog that's focused on the gourmet side of the cannabis industry. The Herb Somm was created in March 2017 with the goal of educating consumers and the public about culinary cannabis, and healthy ways to incorporate herbal products into everyday life. While there is an emphasis on cannabis pairings and recipes, wellness and CBD education are also a focus.

—Jamie Evans, Founder

Visit *TheHerbSomm.com*

bibliography

Barrell, Amanda. "Health Benefits of Elderberry." *Medical News Today*, October 9, 2018. https://www.medicalnewstoday.com/articles/323288.

Bartlett, Lindsey. "Cannabis Sales in California Reach $4.4 Billion in 2020: 'Essential,' Edibles, and the Election." *Forbes,* January 29, 2021. https://www.forbes.com/sites /lindseybartlett/2021/01/29/cannabis-sales-in-california-reach-44-billion-in-2020 -essential-edibles-and-the-election.

Bourque, Andre. "How Hemp and the Farm Bill May Change Life as You Know It." *Forbes,* December 17, 2018. https://www.forbes.com/sites/andrebourque/2018/12/17 /how-hemp-and-the-farm-bill-may-change-life-as-you-know-it.

Brand, E. Joseph, and Zhongzhen Zhao. "Cannabis in Chinese Medicine: Are Some Traditional Indications Referenced in Ancient Literature Related to Cannabinoids?" U.S. National Library of Medicine, March 10, 2017. https://www.ncbi.nlm.nih.gov/pmc /articles/PMC5345167.

ChefSteps. "Pâte de Fruit." Accessed December 23, 2021. https://www.chefsteps.com /activities/pate-de-fruit.

DiLonardo, Mary Jo. "CBD vs. THC: What's the Difference?" WebMD, August 18, 2021. https://www.webmd.com/pain-management/cbd-thc-difference.

Evans, Jamie. *Cannabis Drinks: Secrets to Crafting CBD and THC Beverages at Home.* Beverley, MA: Fair Winds Press, 2021.

Evans, Jamie. *The Ultimate Guide to CBD: Explore the World of Cannabidiol; Recipes for Self-Care, Beverages, Cooking, and More.* Beverley, MA: Fair Winds Press, 2020.

Gritzer, Daniel. "Clarified Butter Recipe." Serious Eats, April 17, 2020. https://www .seriouseats.com/clarified-butter-recipe.

Gumbiner, Jann. "History of Cannabis in Ancient China." *Psychology Today*, May 10, 2011. https://www.psychologytoday.com/us/blog/the-teenage-mind/201105/history -cannabis-in-ancient-china.

Hua, Stephanie, and Coreen Carroll. *Edibles: Small Bites for the Modern Cannabis Kitchen.* San Francisco, CA: Chronicle Books, 2018.

Jikomes, Nick. "How to Assess THC and CBD Levels in Cannabis." CeresMED, January 26, 2018. https://ceresmedvt.com/assess-thc-cbd-levels-cannabis-strains-products.

Kanchwala, Hussain. "How Is Gummy Candy Made?" ScienceABC, November 21, 2021. https://www.scienceabc.com/eyeopeners/gummy-candy-made.html.

Konen, Brett. "Dosing Homemade Cannabis Edibles: Why It's Nearly Impossible to Calculate Potency." Leafly, April 10, 2016. https://www.leafly.com/news/science-tech /dosing-homemade-cannabis-edibles-why-its-nearly-impossible-to-cal.

Lange, Caroline. "Everything You Should Know about Agar-Agar—& How to Cook with It." July 1, 2021. https://food52.com/blog/17465-agar-agar-is-inconsistent-wily-mysterious-but-here-s-what-we-know.

Last Prisoner Project. "Policy & Legislative Advocacy." Accessed December 23, 2021. https://www.lastprisonerproject.org/policy-and-advocacy.

Lindsay, Shanel. "6 Decarboxylation Myths: Decarb Weed without False Facts." Ardent Cannabis, November 30, 2019. https://ardentcannabis.com/blog/decarboxylation-myths.

Lindsay, Shanel. "The Ardent Guide to Cannasugar." Ardent Cannabis, March 19, 2021. https://ardentcannabis.com/blog/the-ardent-guide-to-cannasugar.

Lindsay, Shanel. "CBGA Everclear Infusion." Ardent Cannabis, March 19, 2020. https://ardentcannabis.com/blog/cbga-everclear-infusion.

Lindsay, Shanel. "How to Make Cannabis Infused Oil." Ardent Cannabis, August 16, 2018. https://ardentcannabis.com/blog/how-to-infuse-cannabis.

Lo, Monica. "How to Sous Weed." *Sous Weed*, July 13, 2021. https://www.sousweed.com/blog/howtosousweed.

Lo, Monica. "Kief Honey." *Sous Weed*, July 8, 2015. https://www.sousweed.com/blog/2015/7/8/kief-honey.

Macropoulos, Katherine. "How Are Gummy Bears Made?" eHow. Accessed December 23, 2021. https://www.ehow.com/how-does_4886418_how-gummy-bears-made.html.

Marley, Cedella. *Cooking with Herb: 75 Recipes for the Marley Natural Lifestyle.* New York: Penguin Random House, 2017.

Pacific Pectin, Inc. "Technical Information." Accessed December 23, 2021. https://pacificpectin.com/technical-information.

Prohibition Partners. "The Asian Cannabis Report." Prohibition Partners, May 2019. https://prohibitionpartners.com/reports/the-asian-cannabis-report.

Ramage, Cory. "Why and How to Use Lecithin in Baking and Cooking." Fast Easy Bread, December 30, 2018. https://fasteasybread.com/why-and-how-to-use-lecithin-in-baking-and-cooking.

Schaneman, Bart. "Edibles Outperform Cannabis Industry Growth in 2020 on COVID-Spurred Sales Surge." *MJBizDaily,* January 11, 2021. https://mjbizdaily.com/edibles-outperform-cannabis-industry-growth-in-2020-on-covid-spurred-sales-surge.

Sulak, Dustin. "Edibles Dosage Chart: How Strong Is Your Cannabis-Infused Edible?" Leafly, March 2, 2020. https://www.leafly.com/news/cannabis-101/cannabis-edibles-dosage-guide-chart.

Veriheal. "Edible Dosage Calculator: Infusing Your Food with THC & CBD." Veriheal. Accessed December 23, 2021. https://www.veriheal.com/edible-dosage-calculator.

recipe index

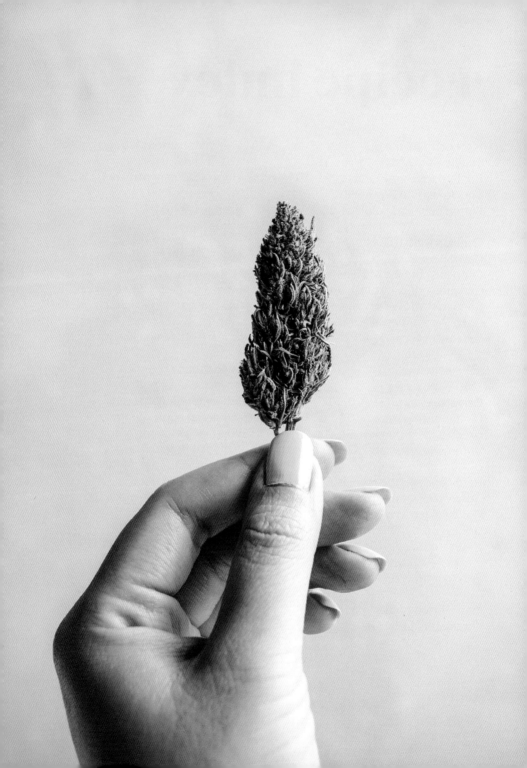

conversions

Volume		
U.S.	**Equivalent**	**Metric**
1 tablespoon (3 teaspoons)	½ fluid ounce	15 milliliters
¼ cup	2 fluid ounces	60 milliliters
⅓ cup	3 fluid ounces	90 milliliters
½ cup	4 fluid ounces	120 milliliters
⅔ cup	5 fluid ounces	150 milliliters
¾ cup	6 fluid ounces	180 milliliters
1 cup	8 fluid ounces	240 milliliters

Weight	
U.S.	**Metric**
1 ounce	30 grams
2 ounces	60 grams
¼ pound	115 grams
⅓ pound	150 grams
½ pound	225 grams
¾ pound	350 grams
1 pound	450 grams

Temperature	
Fahrenheit (°F)	**Celsius (°C)**
120°F	50°C
140°F	60°C
160°F	70°C
180°F	80°C
200°F	95°C
220°F	105°C
240°F	115°C
260°F	125°C
280°F	140°C
300°F	150°C
325°F	165°C
350°F	175°C

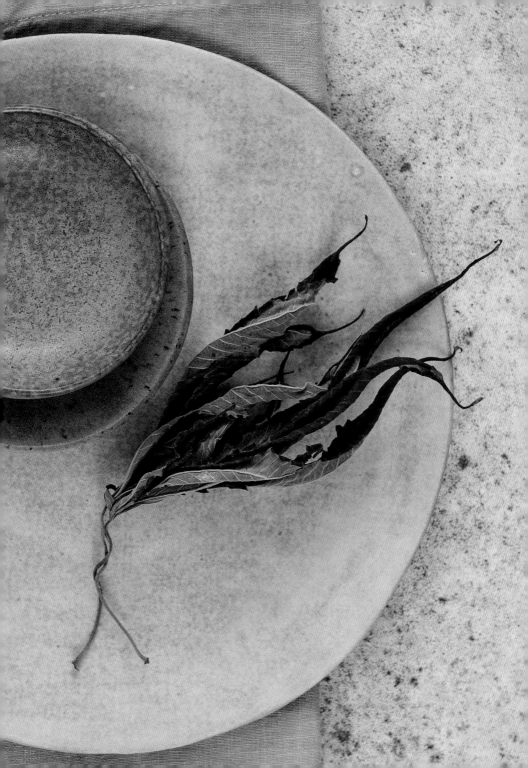

acknowledgments

My heart bursts for my sweet David, Milo, and Starbie. Thank you for providing me with a loving and nurturing environment as I juggle work, life, passion projects, and pregnancy.

Thank you to Mom and Dad for instilling in me such a strong love of food and culture. I appreciate all the encouragement and excitement, especially as we worked on the Taiwanese Nougats together.

To Scott Peabody, Patrick Wong, and June Lee, my best food friends whom I lovingly call my *crumb dumpsters*—thank you for lending your highly critical taste buds and culinary savvy during recipe testing. Our group chat gives me so much life.

Thanks to Ingrid Goesnar, Haejin Chun, and Courtney Wu for gassing me up and all the full belly laughs in a time of immense change and uncertainty. There's no way I could have survived the past few years without our catch-up sessions.

Jamie Evans, your sage advice and impressive organizational pro-tips set me up for success as I set off on this book journey. Lily Bussel—your expertise, enthusiasm, and eyeballs were so appreciated. Thank you both for your willingness to share your talents with me.

A special thank you to Casie Vogel, Renee Rutledge, Claire Chun, and the wonderful team at Ulysses Press for giving this Virgo all the creative freedom she needs to thrive.

Finally, my sincerest gratitude to all the readers and followers of *Sous Weed*. Please know that your support throughout these years has been a fire within me. It has been the most rewarding experience and I so appreciate you all.

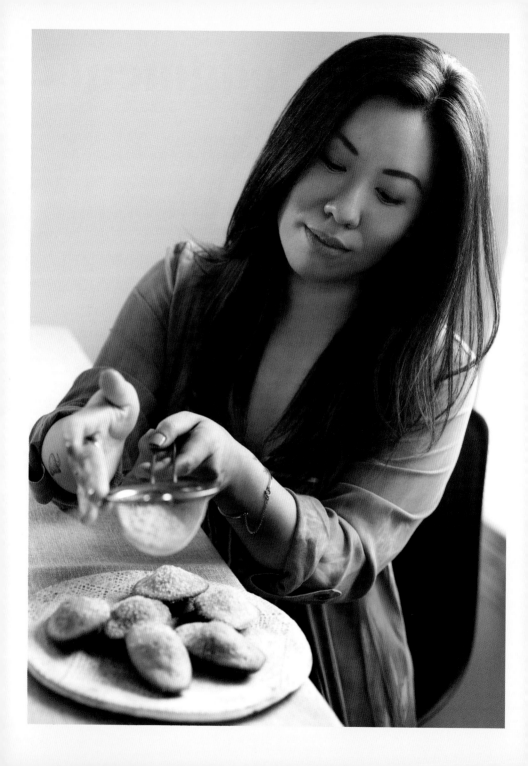

about the author

Monica Lo is a multidisciplinary creative and the creator of *Sous Weed*, a blog turned culinary-cannabis resource founded in 2015. With a formal background in communication design from Pratt Institute, she honed her skills as a food photographer and stylist while working in the advertising industry in New York City.

Her work for *Sous Weed* has been featured on *The Today Show*, VICE's Munchies, Healthyish, and in magazines such as *Vogue* and *Kitchen Toke*. Born in Dallas to food-loving Taiwanese immigrants, she finds pleasure in documenting family recipes for posterity, collecting vintage Chinese cookbooks, and researching ancestral cannabis in ancient Asia.

Monica currently resides in San Francisco with her husband, son, and beloved chihuahua.

To learn more, visit sousweed.com.

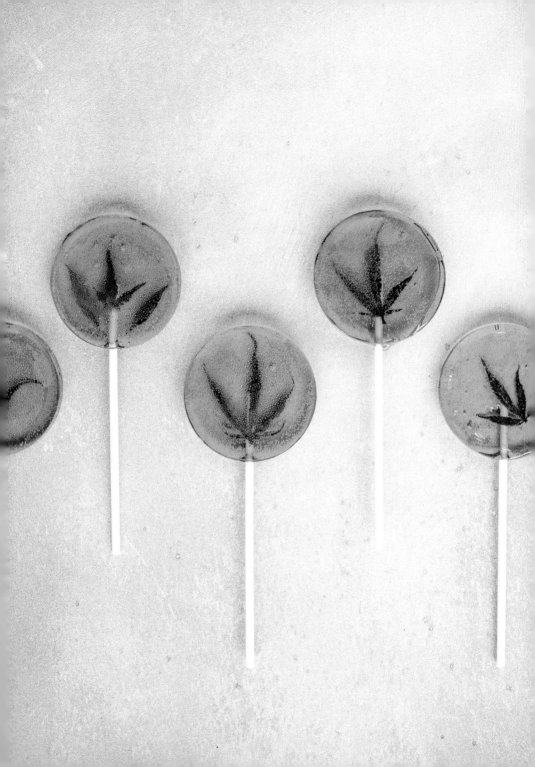